BIOCHEMISTRY LABORATORY PRACTICAL MANUAL
FOR
PHASE-I MBBS STUDENTS

STUDENT NAME: _____

COLLEGE NAME: _____

ROLL NO.: _____ UNIVERSITY EXAM NO.: _____

YEAR: _____ BATCH: _____

BIOCHEMISTRY LABORATORY PRACTICAL MANUAL FOR PHASE-I MBBS STUDENTS

As per the Competency-Based Medical Education Curriculum (NMC)

SECOND EDITION

Pankaja Naik PhD
Professor
Department of Biochemistry
SMBT Institute of Medical Sciences and Research Center
Nashik, Maharashtra, India

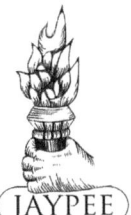

JAYPEE BROTHERS MEDICAL PUBLISHERS
The Health Sciences Publisher
New Delhi | London

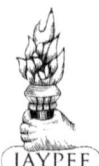 **Jaypee Brothers Medical Publishers (P) Ltd.**

Headquarters

Jaypee Brothers Medical Publishers (P) Ltd
EMCA House, 23/23-B
Ansari Road, Daryaganj
New Delhi 110 002, India
Landline: +91-11-23272143, +91-11-23272703
+91-11-23282021, +91-11-23245672
Email: jaypee@jaypeebrothers.com

Overseas Office

J.P. Medical Ltd
83 Victoria Street, London
SW1H 0HW (UK)
Phone: +44 20 3170 8910
Email: info@jpmedpub.com

Corporate Office

Jaypee Brothers Medical Publishers (P) Ltd
4838/24, Ansari Road, Daryaganj
New Delhi 110 002, India
Phone: +91-11-43574357
Fax: +91-11-43574314
Email: jaypee@jaypeebrothers.com

EU GPSR Authorised Representative

Logos Europe, 9 rue Nicolas Poussin
17000, La Rochelle, France
Phone: +33 (0) 6 67 93 73 78
E-mail: Contact@logoseurope.eu

Website: www.jaypeebrothers.com
Website: www.jaypeedigital.com

© 2024, Jaypee Brothers Medical Publishers

The views and opinions expressed in this book are solely those of the original contributor(s)/author(s) and do not necessarily represent those of editor(s) and publisher of the book.

All rights reserved. No part of this publication may be reproduced, stored or transmitted in any form or by any means, electronic, mechanical, photocopying, recording or otherwise, without the prior permission in writing of the publishers.

All brand names and product names used in this book are trade names, service marks, trademarks or registered trademarks of their respective owners. The publisher is not associated with any product or vendor mentioned in this book.

Medical knowledge and practice change constantly. This book is designed to provide accurate, authoritative information about the subject matter in question. However, readers are advised to check the most current information available on procedures included and check information from the manufacturer of each product to be administered, to verify the recommended dose, formula, method and duration of administration, adverse effects and contraindications. It is the responsibility of the practitioner to take all appropriate safety precautions. Neither the publisher nor the author(s)/editor(s) assume any liability for any injury and/or damage to persons or property arising from or related to use of material in this book.

This book is sold on the understanding that the publisher is not engaged in providing professional medical services. If such advice or services are required, the services of a competent medical professional should be sought.

Every effort has been made where necessary to contact holders of copyright to obtain permission to reproduce copyright material. If any have been inadvertently overlooked, the publisher will be pleased to make the necessary arrangements at the first opportunity.

Inquiries for bulk sales may be solicited at: jaypee@jaypeebrothers.com

Biochemistry Laboratory Practical Manual for Phase-I MBBS Students

First Edition: 2023

Second Edition: **2024**

ISBN: 978-93-5696-379-5

Certificate

Department of Biochemistry

Name of the College: _____

_____

This is to certify that Mr/Ms_____

Roll No. _____ has satisfactorily carried out the practical work in Biochemistry as prescribed for 1st MBBS Examination.

1st Internal Assessment: _____

2nd Internal Assessment: _____

3rd Internal Assessment: _____

Head of the Department   **External Examiner**

Contents

Ex. No.	Experiment	Competency	Page No.	Date	Sign
	Section A: SGD/Demo				
1.	Commonly Used Lab Apparatus: Glassware and Equipment		3		
2.	Good and Safe Lab Practices	BI11.1	12		
3.	Biomedical Waste Management in Lab		17		
4.	Sample Collection		22		
5.	Quality Control	BI11.16	29		
6.	pH Meter and Preparation of Buffers	BI11.2 BI11.16 BI11.19	37		
7.	Principles of Colorimetry and Spectrophotometer	BI11.6 BI11.18 BI11.19	43		
8.	Electrolyte Analysis by Ion Selective Electrode (ISE)		51		
9.	Enzyme-linked Immunosorbent Assay (ELISA)		56		
10.	Immunodiffusion		63		
11.	DNA Isolation from blood/tissues	BI11.16	68		
12.	Autoanalyzer	BI11.19	73		
13.	Protein Electrophoresis and PAGE		79		
14.	Paper Chromatography of Amino Acids and TLC		88		
15.	Arterial Blood Gas (ABG) Analyzer		95		
16.	Composition of CSF	BI11.15	101		
	Section B: Qualitative Experiments (DOAP/SGD)				
17.	Physical and Chemical Components of Normal Urine and Analysis of Normal Urine	BI11.3 BI11.4	111		
18.	Physical and Chemical Components and Analysis of Abnormal Urine and Interpretation	BI11.4 BI11.20	120		
19.	Screening of Urine for Inborn Errors and the Use of Paper Chromatography	BI11.5	137		
	Section C: Quantitative Experiments (Practical/DOAP)				
20.	Estimation of Blood Glucose		145		
21.	Estimation of Blood Urea	BI11.21	153		
22.	Estimation of Serum and urine Creatinine and Creatinine Clearance	BI11.7 BI11.22	159		

Ex. No.	Experiment	Competency	Page No.	Date	Sign
23.	Estimation of Serum Proteins, Albumin and A:G Ratio	BI11.8 BI11.21 BI11.22	168		
24.	Estimation of Serum Calcium	BI11.11	176		
25.	Estimation of Serum Phosphorous		182		
26.	Estimation of Serum Bilirubin	BI11.12	188		
27.	Estimation of Serum Transaminases (SGPT/ALT and SGOT/AST)	BI11.13	195		
28.	Estimation of Serum Alkaline Phosphatase	BI11.14	203		
29.	Estimation of Serum Total Cholesterol	BI11.9	209		
30.	Estimation of Serum HDL Cholesterol		215		
31.	Estimation of Serum Triglycerides	BI11.10	221		
Section D: Basis and Rationale of Biochemical Tests Done in Various Disorders (SGD)					
32.	Basis and Rationale of Biochemical Tests Done in Various Disorders:				
	Diabetes Mellitus		229		
	Dyslipidemia		230		
	Myocardial Infarction		231		
	Liver Disease, Jaundice		232		
	Pancreatitis		233		
	Nephrotic Syndrome	BI11.17	234		
	Proteinuria		235		
	Edema		237		
	Renal Failure		237		
	Gout		240		
	Thyroid Disorders		240		
	Acid-Base Balance		241		

DOAP: Demonstrate, Observe, Assess, and Perform; SGD: Small Group Discussion

General/Safety Biochemistry Lab Rules and Guidelines

It is each student's responsibility to read and understand all of the biochemistry lab rules and guidelines.

1. Students need to be on time
2. Lab coat and shoes are compulsory during practicals.
3. Hair must be tied up (especially girls) before entering the laboratory.
4. Cell phone use is not permitted in the labs as students need to be focused on their lab work for safety reasons
5. Follow all instructions given by your teacher.
6. Conduct yourself in a responsible and professional manner at all times.
7. Make separate notebook for biochemistry practical. Enter your observations, calculations and results in a systematic way.
8. Label all your test tubes properly.
9. Show your results to the batch teacher and get it signed.
10. Students need to perform with caution in the laboratory as they may work with potentially hazardous chemical and agents, as well as open flames.
11. Strong acids/alkalis should not be mouth pipetted, instead use dispensers, pipette pump or micropipettes.
12. Take extreme care while pipetting, heating & handling corrosive reagents.
13. For any help required regarding chemicals, glassware, reagents, samples, etc., contact the technicians present in the laboratory.
14. Put off the burners when not in use.
15. Students are required to clean their workspace before leaving the labs. That includes placing all materials back into their proper place, washing of glassware, discarding lab waste into the proper containers, pushing chairs in, removing all trash and washing hands.
16. No eating or drinking is allowed in the laboratories or prep rooms. All drinks and food items (including chewing gum) need to be left outside the labs.
17. Students need to be aware and alert at all times in the lab, and their focus needs to be on the lab work.
18. Any personal business, such as talking on the phone and/or texting, will not be tolerated in lab/during lab time.
19. Look for announcements on noticeboard regularly.
20. Students are required to work independently and submit their own, original work.

SECTION A

SGD/Demo

Section Outline

Experiment 1: Commonly Used Lab Apparatus: Glassware and Equipment
Experiment 2: Good and Safe Lab Practices
Experiment 3: Biomedical Waste Management in Lab
Experiment 4: Sample Collection
Experiment 5: Quality Control
Experiment 6: pH Meter and Preparation of Buffers
Experiment 7: Principles of Colorimetry and Spectrophotometer
Experiment 8: Electrolyte Analysis by Ion Selective Electrode
Experiment 9: Enzyme-Linked Immunosorbent Assay
Experiment 10: Immunodiffusion
Experiment 11: DNA Isolation from Blood/Tissues
Experiment 12: Autoanalyzer
Experiment 13: Protein Electrophoresis and PAGE
Experiment 14: Paper Chromatography of Amino Acids and TLC
Experiment 15: Arterial Blood Gas (ABG) Analyzer
Experiment 16: Composition of CSF

EXPERIMENT 1

Commonly Used Lab Apparatus: Glassware and Equipment

COMPETENCY	LEARNING OBJECTIVES
BI11.1 Describe commonly used laboratory apparatus and equipment, good safe laboratory practice and waste disposal.	1. Describe commonly used apparatus in the laboratory and their use. 2. Describe commonly used equipments in the laboratory and their use.

INTRODUCTION

There are varieties of apparatus and equipments which are being used in biochemistry laboratory for teaching and diagnostic purposes. The commonly used apparatus and equipments are given below. It is essential to understand the functioning of these apparatus and equipments, as ineffectiveness not only increases the risk of experimental error but also poses a potential laboratory hazard. The following are the commonly used biochemistry lab apparatus and equipments, along with their uses.

COMMONLY USED APPARATUS AND THEIR USE

The commonly used apparatus in the biochemistry laboratory include:

Beakers

Beakers are cylindrical, have a flat bottom, and a small spout on the top to pour chemicals. Beakers are usually made of borosilicate glass. They also commonly have markings to measure the volume they contain, although they are not a precise way to measure liquids. Beakers come in several sizes **(Figure 1.1)** with volumes ranging from 5 milliliters to 10,000 milliliters. Beakers are used for mixing, stirring, and heating chemicals. They are mostly used for the preparation of various solutions.

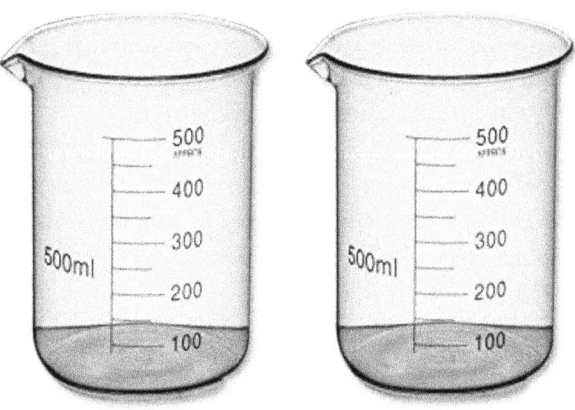

Figure 1.1: Beakers.

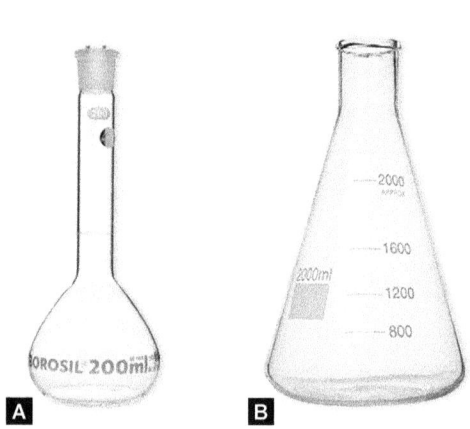

Figures 1.2A and B: Volumetric and conical flasks: (A) Volumetric flask; (B) Conical flask.

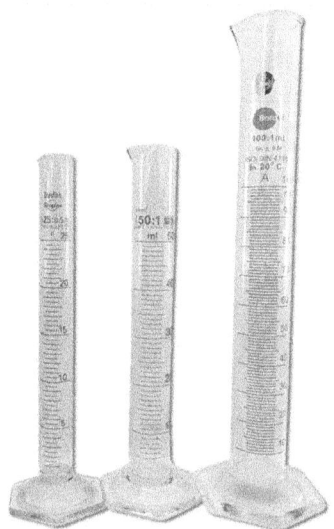

Figure 1.3: Measuring cylinder.

Flasks

They come in a variety of shapes and sizes, with each one having a specific purpose associated with it. Various types of flasks are conical, volumetric (**Figures 1.2A and B**), flat bottomed or round bottomed flasks.
- **Conical flask** also known as Erlenmeyer flask is one of the most commonly used flasks to carry out various experiments in the biochemistry lab, such as titration, filtration, crystallization, etc. It has a narrow neck and expands toward its base. This allows easy mixing and swirling of the flask without too much risk of spilling.
- A **volumetric flask** is one of the laboratory glassware primarily used to prepare solutions. They are used to make the final volume of the solution accurately. They have a capacity from 25 to 5000 mL.

Measuring Cylinders

Just as the name suggests, this glassware is cylindrical and is used to measure the volume of a liquid. It is graduated, and every marking shows the amount of a reagent. They have a capacity from 10 to 2000 mL (**Figure 1.3**). They are used to measure the volume of the liquid.

Reagent Bottles

The reagent bottles are used to store chemicals in liquid or powder form for laboratories and stored in cabinets or on shelves. They usually have white or brown glass (**Figure 1.4**)

Pipettes

These are used for dispensing specific quantities of liquids. The following are the pipettes used in the clinical chemistry laboratory **(Figures 1.5A to D).**
- **Graduated pipettes:** They are available from 0.1 mL to 10 mL. The graduations are durable and resistant to chemical attack and normal washings.
- **Autopipettes:** A mechanical pipette that can transfer measured amounts of a liquid automatically. Unlike manual pipetting, **there is a decrease in human errors because the machines carry out all the manual work.** The autopipette allows rapid

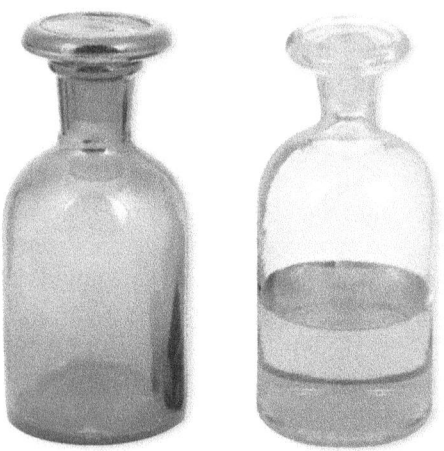

Figure 1.4: Reagent bottles.

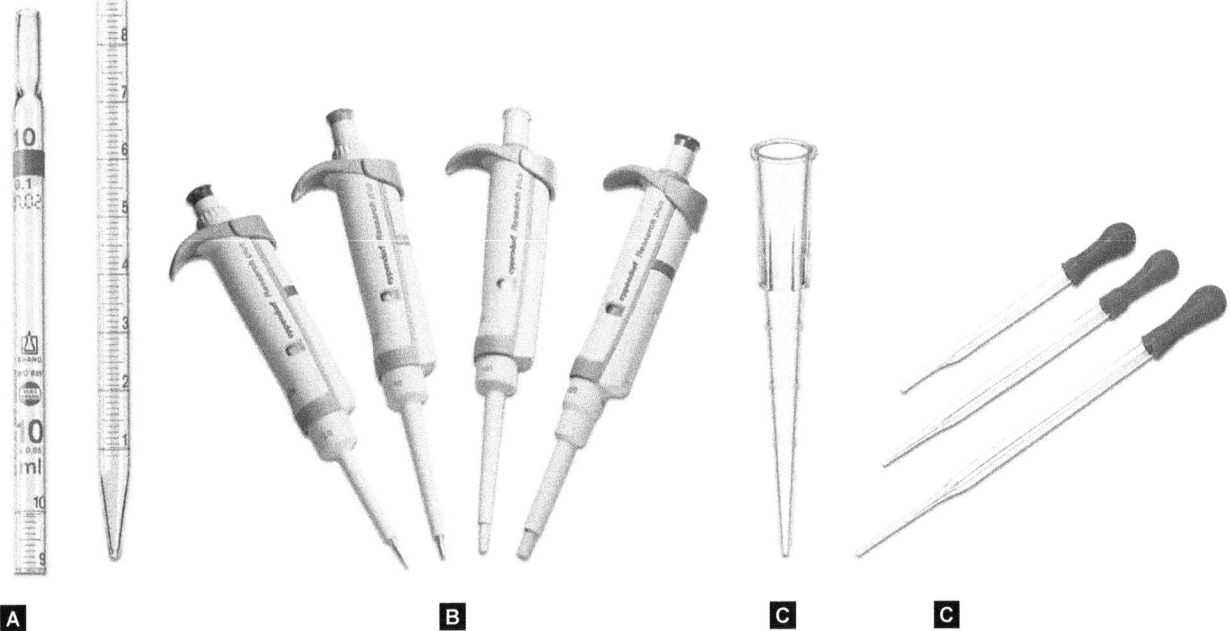

Figures 1.5A to D: Types of pipette: (A) Graduated pipette; (B) Autopipette; (C) Autopipette tip; (D) Pasture pipette.

and accurate dispensing of measured volumes of liquid ranging from 1 to 1000 microliters. They allow the selection of a volume within the given range. The disposable tips are used in these pipettes.They are used in molecular and clinical chemistry laboratory. The automated pipetting provides increased reproducibility in the laboratory. That means the technique helps obtain consistent results. The machines carry out all the work, and the contamination decreases.

- **Pasture pipette:** A pasture pipette, sometimes known as a dropper, is used in biochemistry labs to transfer extremely small quantities of liquids. They have a compressible bulb on the top that aids in the flow of the liquid.

Pipette Pump

Pipette pump is a fast release pipetting device for precise pipetting **(Figure 1.6)**. Pipette pumps contains a rotating thumb wheel which provides safe and accurate pipetting and dispensing of reagents from graduated pipettes. It can be used to deliver measured volume of reagents ranging from 1 to 10 mL.

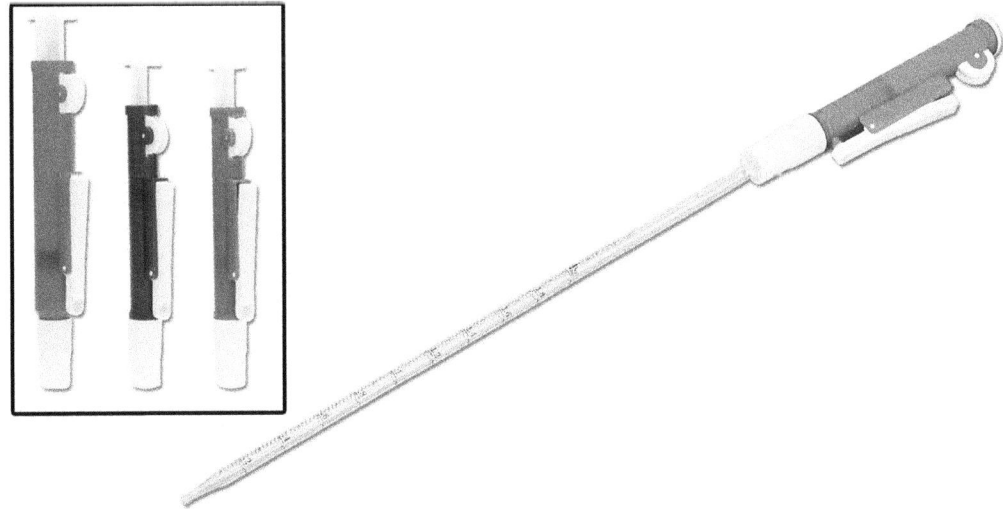

Figure 1.6: Pipette pump.

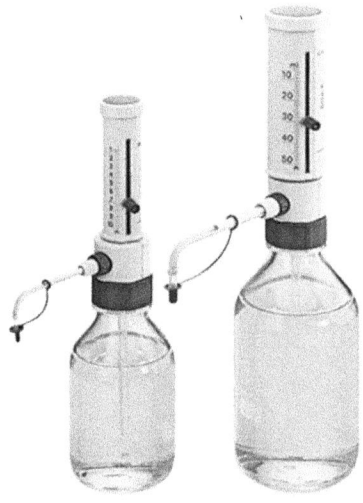
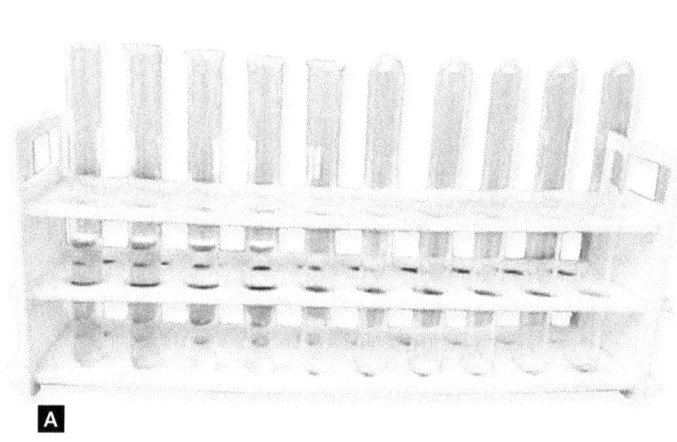

Figure 1.7: Bottle dispenser.

Figures 1.8A and B: Test tubes: (A) Test tubes with test tube stand; (B) Centrifuge tubes.

Bottle Dispenser

A bottle dispenser is used to dispense precise amounts of chemical reagents from bottles **(Figure 1.7)**. Bottle dispensers can safely dispense a fixed amount of liquid usually between 1 mL and 100 mL, directly from a bottle. Bottle dispensers help to reduce the loss of reagents, save time and increases work efficiency.

Test Tubes

The test tubes are commonly used in various biochemistry tests. They are primarily used for qualitative assessment. It is used to hold chemicals during the experiments. Due to their high thermal stability, test tubes can be used to heat or boil chemical samples. While heating, it is essential to hold the test tube at a 45° angle so that the gases formed inside the narrow tube may easily escape without causing the hot liquid to shoot up. They are generally held in a test tube rack specifically designed for the purpose **(Figures 1.8A and B)**

Centrifuge tubes are either graduated or plain and are available in conical shape. They are used in a centrifuge machine to separate the components of solutions.

Test Tube Holder

A test tube holder is a device used to hold test tubes while heating them **(Figure 1.9)**. It provides a safe distance between the person's hand and the test tube, protecting the skin from accidental burns caused by the spilling of chemicals.

Wash Bottle

The wash bottle is a regular plastic bottle attached to a nozzle with a screw-top lid **(Figure 1.10)**, and it is used to rinse various pieces of laboratory glassware, such as test tubes and round bottom flasks, after or before their use.

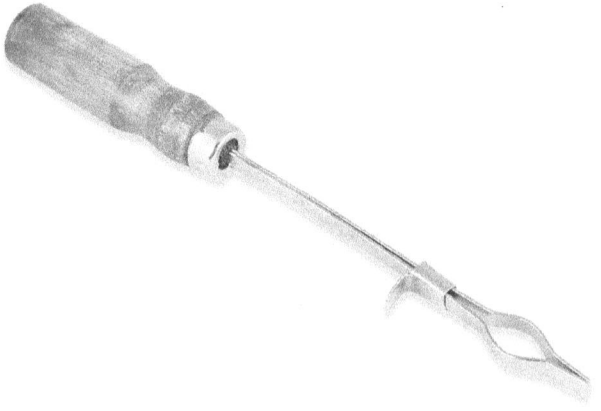

Figure 1.9: Test tube holder.

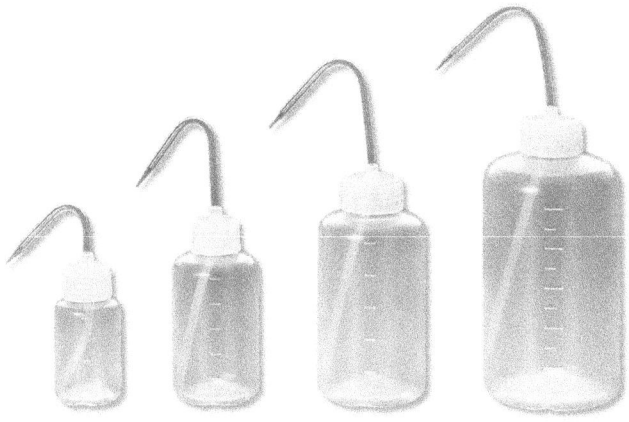

Figure 1.10: Wash bottle.

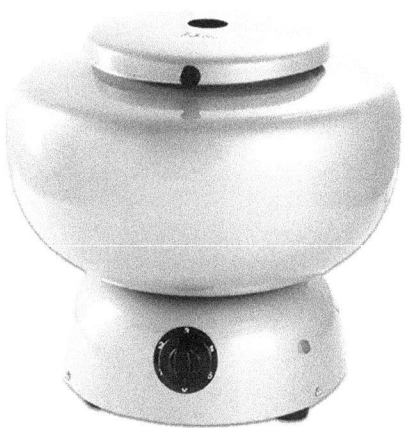

Figure 1.11: Centrifuge machine.

COMMONLY USED EQUIPMENTS AND THEIR USE

Centrifuge

A centrifuge is **a device that uses centrifugal force to separate various components of a fluid (Figure 1.11)**. This is achieved by spinning the fluid at high speed within a container, thereby separating fluids of different densities or liquids from solids.

Uses

- The separation of plasma from whole blood or serum from clotted blood
- Separation of sediments in urine

Water Bath

The water bath is used to maintain the temperature required to carry out various chemical reactions at specific temperature (**Figure 1.12**). The temperature of the water bath is controlled by a thermostatic arrangement.

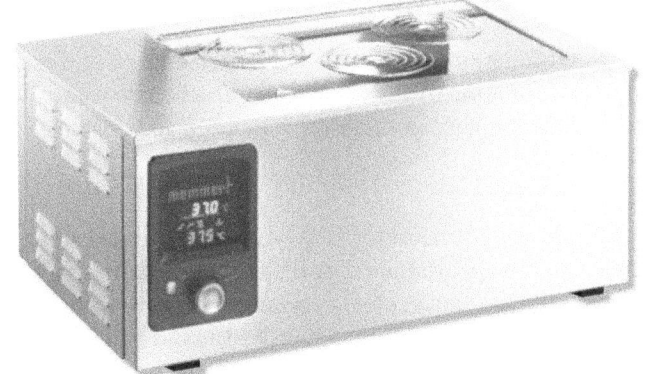

Figure 1.12: Water bath.

Uses

A water bath is used **to incubate samples at a constant temperature for the** determination of:
- Serum enzymes at 37°C
- Glucose, urea, cholesterol, triglycerides, etc., at 37°C

Hot Air Oven

It uses dry heat to sterilize laboratory equipment and other materials (**Figure 1.13**). Generally, they use a thermostat to control the temperature. The temperature may go up to 250°C.

This is used for:
- Dry sterilization in microbiological experiments
- Heating of chemicals wherever required
- Drying of chemicals, e.g., preparation of anticoagulated bulbs
- Drying of glassware

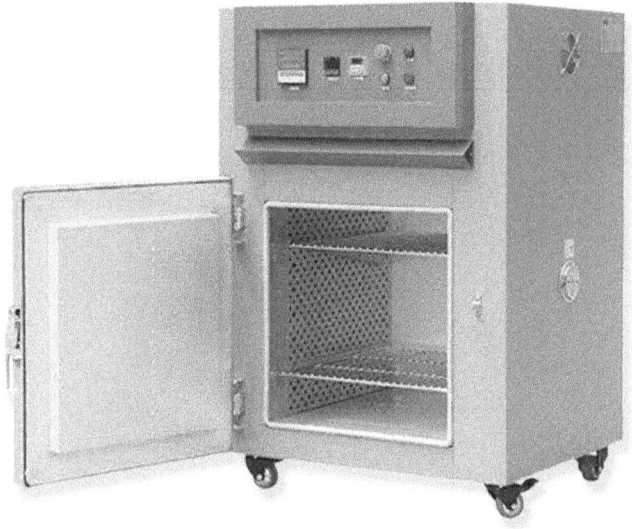

Figure 1.13: Hot air oven.

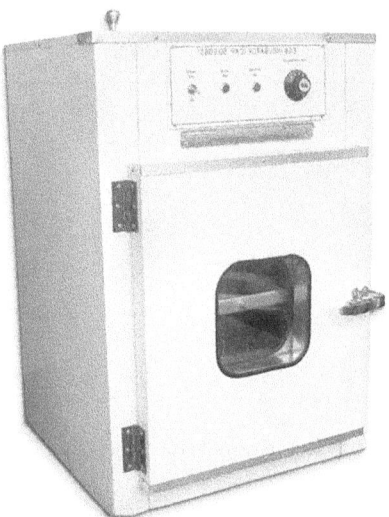

Figure 1.14: Incubator.

Incubator

It is a heated, insulated box used to grow microbiological or cell cultures. The laboratory incubator does this by maintaining optimal temperature, humidity, and gaseous content of the atmosphere inside (**Figure 1.14**). It provides temperature between 6–70°C. The incubator has a wide range of use. Some of the applications are as follows:
- Determination of enzymes in the specimen by end point reaction methods.
- Determination of glucose, urea, uric acid, cholesterol, triglycerides, etc., by enzymatic methods.
- In microbiology laboratories, it helps to grow bacteria, fungi, and other microorganisms

Colorimeter

A laboratory colorimeter is an instrument used to measure the absorbance of wavelengths of light at a particular frequency (color) by a sample (**Figure 1.15**)

Digital colorimeters are widely used across different work areas including, environmental testing, clinical diagnostics, pharmaceutical analysis, and biochemistry. Laboratory colorimeters are used to determine the concentration of a known solute in a sample since the concentration of a solute is proportional to the absorbance.

Uses of Colorimeter

- The colorimeter is commonly used for the determination of the concentration of a colored compound by measuring the optical density or its absorbance.
- Colorimeters are frequently used in the medicine to estimate biochemical samples, such as blood, urine, cerebral spinal fluid, plasma, serum, and so on.

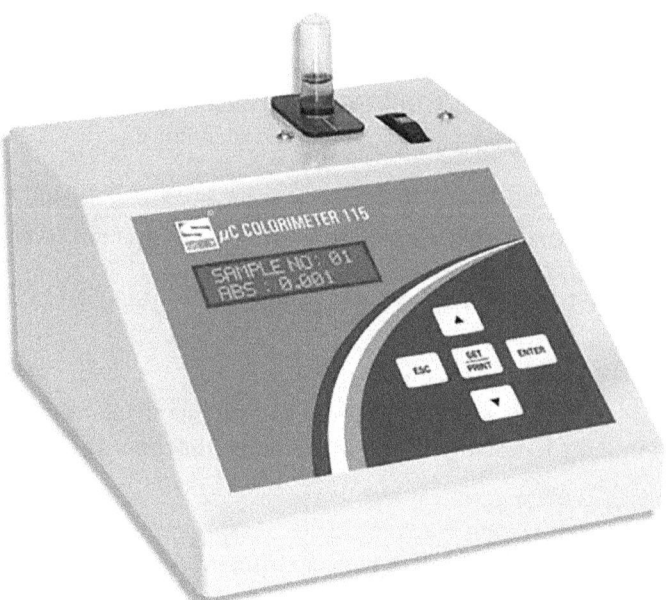

Figure 1.15: Digital colorimeter.

pH Meter

pH meter is an instrument used to measure pH of a solution **(Figure 1.16)**. In the laboratory, pH meters are used to measure the pH of various chemical solutions in research and quality control applications.

AUTOANALYZER

Semi-autoanalyzers

Semi-automatic biochemistry analyzer is capable of performing routine biochemistry, hormonal assay, electrolytes, and enzyme investigations **(Figure 1.17)**. This instrument is based on principle colorimetric analysis.

Semi-auto biochemistry analyzer is capable to perform tests on whole blood, serum, plasma, cerebrospinal fluid and urine as sample.

Fully Automated Biochemistry Analyzer

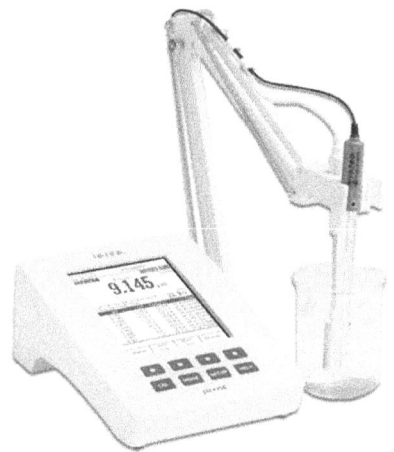

Figure 1.16: pH meter.

Fully automated analyzer is a medical laboratory instrument designed to measure different chemicals and other characteristics in a number of biological samples quickly, with minimal human assistance which is used for diagnosis of disease. This instrument is based on colorimetric principle **(Figure 1.18)**. computer and robotic technology is used to perform repetitive tasks, such as pipetting, mixing, dispensing, etc.

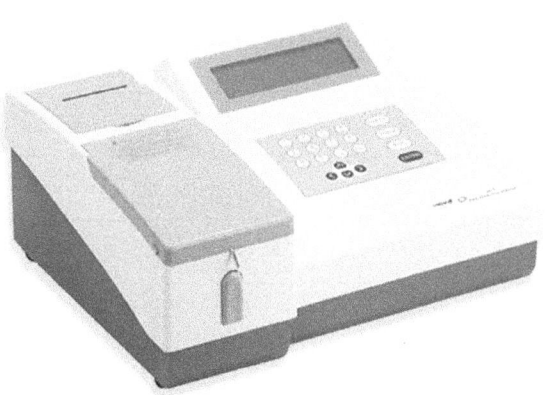

Figure 1.17: Semiautomatic biochemistry analyzer.

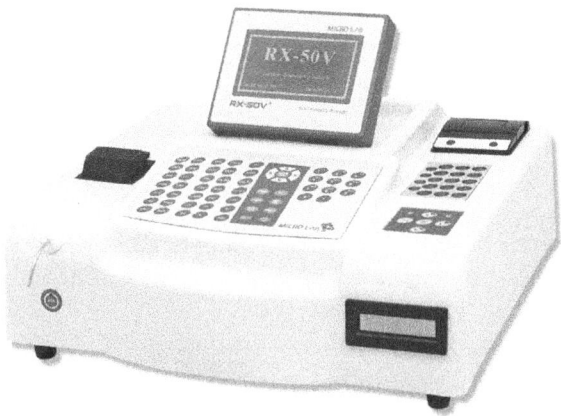

Figure 1.18: Fully automated biochemistry analyzer.

QUESTIONS

1. Write the use of autopipette.
2. Write the use of incubator in laboratory.
3. What are the different types of the pipette? Write their use in laboratory.
4. Write the use of bottle dispenser.
5. Write the use of water bath in laboratory.
6. Write the use of pipette pump.
7. Write the use of test tubes.
8. Enumerate commonly used equipments in the laboratory.
9. Write the use of colorimeter.
10. Write use of fully autoanalyzer.
11. Write use of water bath and hot air oven in laboratory.
12. Write use of pH meter and incubator in laboratory.

EXPERIMENT 2

Good and Safe Lab Practices

COMPETENCY	LEARNING OBJECTIVES
BI11.1 Describe commonly used laboratory apparatus and equipments good safe laboratory practice and waste disposal.	1. Describe safety measures in lab to prevent laboratory hazards.

INTRODUCTION

All clinical laboratory persons are constantly exposed to various hazards, such as electric shock, radioactive material hazard, gaseous hazard, corrosive substances and risk of handling biological material. Lab students must well know about the rules and introductions in laboratory, common hazard symbols and their meanings, laboratory emergencies and first aid, personal protective equipment, how to store the chemicals safely and how to act at putting off fire.

Safety is important when working in the lab because it helps you avoid injury, keep yourself from making mistakes and prevents laboratory accidents in the laboratory.

SAFETY MEASURES IN LAB

There are many aspects to the safe operation of a clinical laboratory to prevent laboratory hazards which include:

Personal Safety

- Wear a sensible clothes full covered shoes and safety shield or glasses and wear safety goggles to protect your eyes when heating substances, dissecting, etc.
- Barrier protection, such as gloves and lab coats must be used when handling corrosive substances and patients' specimens.
- If you have long hair or loose clothes, make sure it is tied back or confined.
- Never eat or drink while working in the laboratory
- Make a habit of keeping your hands away from your mouth, nose, eyes and any other mucous membranes to reduce the possibility of self-inoculation.
- Encourage frequent hand washing in the laboratory. Employees must wash their hands whenever they leave the laboratory.

Chemical Safety

- All samples should be considered potentially hazardous and handled accordingly.
- Do not taste or smell chemicals
- Never perform mouth pipetting and never blow out pipettes that contain potentially infectious material.
- All chemicals must be properly labeled and stored in an organized manner. Labels should be kept up-to-date, so that you know what chemicals are being stored in each container. The labels should also tell you about possible hazards associated with the material and instruct you on how to handle it safely.
- All waste materials must be disposed of according to the regulations set by your institution or organization.
- Chemical injuries are commonly encountered following exposure to acids and alkali. In such cases, treat the injury/burn as described:
  - Skin burn should be washed under running water or iced water and apply petroleum jelly or burn ointment and cover with sterile gauze. Ask for medical attention.
  - Chemical injury to eyes must be treated immediately by flushing eyes with water for at least 15 min. the eyes must be forcibly held open to wash and the eyeballs must be rotated so that all the surface area is rinsed and immediately be taken to the ophthalmologist.
  - Inhalation injury by toxic fumes is treated by closing containers, opening windows or otherwise and moving to fresh air. Irritation to throat can be smoothened with hot water vapor inhalation and a warm drink.
  - In accidental swallowing of chemicals, the mouth must be thoroughly rinsed with water. If proper swallowing has occurred, the person should be made to drink water followed by milk in case of acids. In case of alkali lemon juice or dilute vinegar (1:3/vinegar: water) should be given after water.

Biological Safety

- Clinical lab personnel deal with potential infectious blood and other biological samples. Accidental spillage of blood and body fluid may occur during sample collection, sample transport or while the test is being performed. All spillages are considered to be potentially infectious.
- Any infectious material (blood, urine, or any other biological material) if spilled,
  - Flood the area with 1% hypochlorite solution.
  - Cover the area with absorbent material.
  - Duration of contact to be 15–20 minutes.
  - Collect entire material using scoop and scraper and place it in yellow colored BMW bag.
  - Mop the area using detergent.
- Each laboratory/Ward in a hospital handling blood and body fluids should have a spillage tray readily available containing:
  - Protective apron
  - Single-use gloves
  - Surgical mask
  - Eye protection device
  - Scoop and scraper
  - Absorbent material (e.g., cotton roll, tissue paper, newspaper, etc.)
  - Yellow-colored biomedical waste (BMW) bag
  - 1% hypochlorite solution
- Avoid handling needles directly; use needle sheath and dispose of needles in rigid containers to prevent accidental injuries.
- Decontaminate all surfaces and reusable devices after use with appropriate hospital disinfectants.
- Before centrifuging tubes, inspect them for cracks.
- Use biomedical waste management handling rules.
- Never leave a discarded tube or infected material unattended or unlabeled.
- Clean out freezer and dry-ice chests to remove broken ampoules and tubes of biological specimens periodically.

QUESTIONS

1. Write personal safety measures in lab.
2. Write biological safety measures in lab.
3. Write chemical safety measures in lab.
4. What are the steps to be follow in case of accidental spill?
5. Write importance of good and safe lab practices.

EXPERIMENT 3

Biomedical Waste Management in Lab

COMPETENCY	LEARNING OBJECTIVES
BI11.1 Describe commonly used laboratory apparatus and equipment, good safe laboratory practice and waste disposal.	1. Define biomedical waste (BMW). 2. Classify hazardous waste. 3. Describe steps involved in biomedical waste management.

INTRODUCTION

Biomedical waste (BMW) includes all the waste generated from healthcare facility which can have any adverse effect to the health of a person or to the environment in general if not disposed properly.

DEFINITION

Biomedical waste (BMW) means any waste, which is generated during the diagnosis, treatment or immunization of human beings or animals or research activities pertaining to or in the production or testing of biological samples.

CLASSIFICATION OF HAZARDOUS WASTE

About 75 to 90% of the waste produced by healthcare providers is non-hazardous **general waste** comparable to domestic waste. About 20% of the waste is considered hazardous and/or infectious. If segregation does not take place, all the waste produced should be considered as infectious as it is mixed. WHO has classified hazardous waste into following categories:

- **Infectious waste:** (Suspected to contain pathogens), e.g., laboratory culture, waste from isolation
- **Pathological waste:** (Containing human tissue or fluids), e.g., body parts, blood and other body fluids, fetuses
- **Sharps:** (Sharp material), e.g., needles, infusion sets, scalpels, knives, blades, broken glass
- **Pharmaceutical waste:** (Containing pharmaceuticals), e.g., expired drugs, contaminated bottles, boxes
- **Genotoxic waste:** Waste containing cytostatic drugs (drugs used for the treatment of cancer) genotoxic chemicals
- **Chemical waste:** (Substance containing chemical substance), e.g., laboratory reagents, film developer, expired disinfectants, solvents
- **Waste with heavy metals:** Batteries, broken thermometer

❖ **Pressurized containers:** Gas cylinders, gas cartridges, aerosol cans
❖ **Radioactive material:** (Substances containing radioactive substances), e.g., unused liquid from radiotherapy, contaminated glassware, urine, excreta from patient treated with unsealed radionucleotides.

STEPS INVOLVED IN BIOMEDICAL WASTE MANAGEMENT

The various steps involved in the management of biomedical waste are as follows:
❖ **Collection:** It should be collected at the point of generation by a healthcare worker.
❖ **Segregation:** Segregation prevents mixing of infectious waste with non-infectious waste.
❖ **Storage:** Segregated biomedical waste is stored in designated color coded plastic bags/ containers as per BMW management and handling rules 2016 **(Table 3.1)**.
❖ **Pretreatment:** Laboratory and highly infectious waste to be pretreated with 1% hypochlorite solution. The minimum contact period should be 6 minutes.
❖ **Transportation:** Transportation of segregated waste to the central storage area should be carried out in especially designed vehicle with label of biohazard **(Figures 3.1A and B)**
❖ **Treatment:** Biomedical waste shall be treated by one of the following method prior to disposal.
  - *Incineration:* A thermal treatment that leads to complete combustion of waste to render it non-pathogenic.
  - *Wet and dry thermal treatment:* Decontamination by heating with steam under pressure (autoclave) so as to render the biochemical waste non-infectious.
  - *Screw-feed technology:* Dry thermal disinfection process in which waste is shredded and heated in a rotating auger
  - *Chemical disinfection:* Chemicals such as sodium hypochlorite or chlorine dioxide are added to waste to kill or inactivate the pathogens it contents.
  - *Microwave irradiation:* Most organisms are destroyed by heating the waste at frequency of about 2450 MHz and a wavelength of 12.24 cm by means of microwaves.
  - *Land disposal:* If a municipality or medical authority genuinely lacks the means to treat waste before disposal, the use of a landfill has to be regarded as an acceptable disposal route.
  - *Inertization*: Inertization involves mixing biomedical waste with cement and other substances before disposal, in order to minimize the risk of toxic substances contained in the wastes migrating into the surface water or ground water
❖ **Disposal:** Depends on the type of biomedical hazards **(Table 3.1)**.

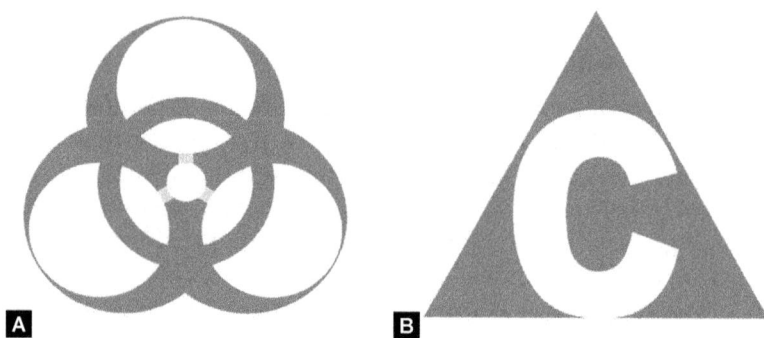

Figures 3.1A and B: The international symbol for biological hazard: (A) Biohazard symbol: (B) Cytotoxic hazard symbol.

Table 3.1: Segregation of biomedical wastes with corresponding color code of containers and their disposal.

Color code	Type of bag/ Container used	Type of waste	Treatment and disposal option
Yellow	Yellow-colored non-chlorinated plastic bag or container	• **Human anatomical waste:** Human tissues, organs, body parts, etc. • **Animal anatomical waste:** Experimental animals' tissues, organs, etc. • **Soiled waste:** Items contaminated with blood, such as cotton swabs, dressings, bags containing residual blood, etc. • **Expired/Discarded medicines:** cytotoxic drugs, items contaminated by cytotoxic drugs, such as glass vials, etc., and antibiotics • **Chemical liquid waste:** Liquid from laboratories, floor washings, etc. • **Contaminated linen:** Mattresses, beddings contaminated with blood or body fluids. • **Microbiology, biotechnology/lab waste:** Blood bags, laboratory cultures, stocks or specimens of microorganisms, attenuated vaccines, human and animal cell cultures used in research or industrial laboratories.	• Incineration or • Plasma pyrolysis or • Deep burial*
Red	Red-colored non-chlorinated plastic bags or containers	**Contaminated waste (recyclable):** Gloves, tubing, syringes, intravenous sets, syringes without needles, vacuum evacuated tubes, etc.	Autoclaving or microwaving/hydroclaving followed by shredding or mutilation. Treated material can be recycled. Plastic waste should not be sent to landfill sites.
White	Puncture-proof, leak-proof, tamper-proof containers	**Waste sharps including metals:** Needles, scalpel, blades, metal sharps, etc.	Autoclaving and dry heat sterilization followed by shredding or mutilation or encapsulation.
Blue	Cardboard boxes with blue-colored marking	**Glassware:** Broken or discarded and contaminated glass including medicine vials and ampoules except those contaminated with cytotoxic wastes. **Metallic body implants**	Disinfection (by soaking the washed glass waste after cleaning with detergent and sodium hypochlorite treatment) or through autoclaving or microwaving or hydroclaving and then sent for recycling

*Disposal by deep burial is permitted only in rural or remote areas where there is no access to common biomedical waste treatment facility. This will be carried out with the prior approval from the prescribed authority and as per the standards.

QUESTIONS

1. What is biomedical waste?
2. Which are the different types of hazardous waste?
3. Write different steps involved in biomedical waste management.
4. Which are the different types of biomedical waste treatment?
5. Write biomedical wastes with corresponding color code of containers as per BMW management and handling rules 2016.

EXPERIMENT 4

Sample Collection

COMPETENCY	LEARNING OBJECTIVES
BI11.1 Describe commonly used laboratory apparatus and equipment, good safe laboratory practice and waste disposal.	1. Describe different types of biological samples. 2. Describe methods of collection of blood sample. 3. Describe color-coded vacuum evacuated tubes, their additives and uses in laboratory. 4. Describe types of urine samples and their collection.

INTRODUCTION

Proper specimen collection and handling is an integral part of obtaining a valid and timely laboratory test result. Specimens must be obtained in the proper tubes or containers, correctly labeled, and then promptly transported to the laboratory.

TYPES OF BIOLOGICAL SAMPLES

Types of biological specimens that are analysed in clinical laboratories include:
- Whole blood
- Serum
- Plasma
- Urine
- Feces
- Various fluids, such as: pleural fluid, ascitic fluid, cerebrospinal fluid (CSF), synovial fluid, pericardial fluid, and amniotic fluid.
    - *Plasma:* Obtained by centrifugation of anticoagulant added blood and it contain all coagulation factors except calcium ions.
    - *Serum:* Obtained when blood undergoes clotting and it does not contain clotting factors.

Among the above, blood and urine are the most common samples analyzed in the laboratory.

METHODS OF BLOOD SAMPLE COLLECTION

Blood samples intended for laboratory analysis are usually collected in glass or plastic tubes that have been partially evacuated so that their internal air pressure is lower than atmospheric pressure. These tubes have color-coded polymer stoppers that indicate their contents.

EXPERIMENT 4: Sample Collection

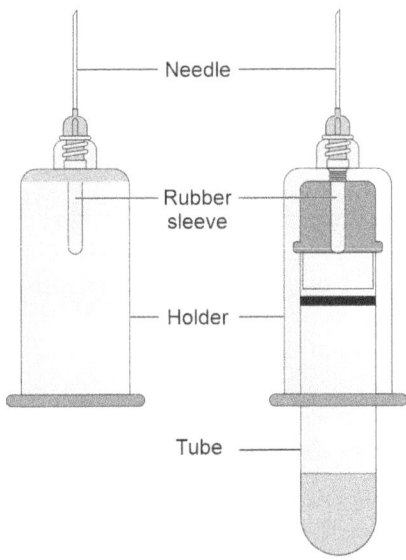

Figure 4.1: Vacuum evacuated tube system.

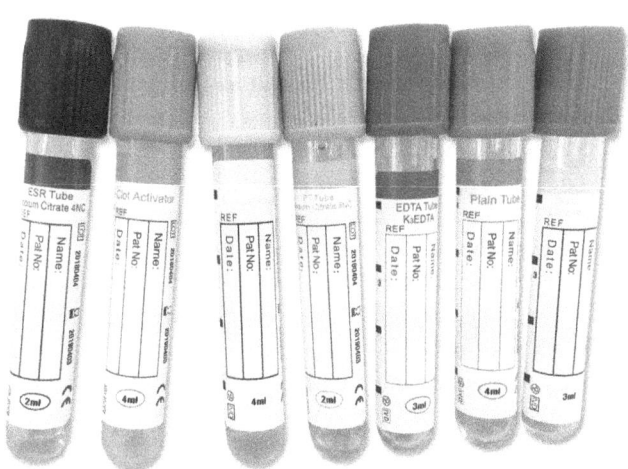

Figure 4.2: Different types of vacuum evacuated tube.

Blood for analysis is collected from **veins, arteries** or **capillaries**. Most of the tests are performed on venous blood, the process of collection of venous blood is called **venipuncture** or **phlebotomy** (from Greek words; **phleb**, which means vein, and **tome**, to cut or incise). Venipuncture can be performed by three basic methods.

1. **Vacuum evacuated tube system:** This system contains a needle, holder, and vacuum tube **(Figure 4.1).** Vacuum evacuated tubes are plastic tubes with color-coded tops indicating tube contents **(Figure 4.2).** Most tubes contain an additive that either accelerates clotting of the blood (clot activator) or prevents the blood from clotting (anticoagulant). They are used to collect blood for various investigation.
2. **Needle and syringe:** Blood collected in a syringe can be transferred to an evacuated tube.
3. **Winged infusion set:** Winged infusion sets are used when blood is collected from a very small vein, e.g., pediatric patient.

ETS is the preferred method. In this method, blood is collected directly from the vein into a tube, minimizing the risk of specimen contamination.

Color-coded Vacuum Evacuated Tubes, their Additives and Uses in Laboratory

Commonly used vacuum evacuated tubes in clinical chemistry lab are **(Table 4.1):**

- **Green top tube:** This less commonly used tube is for biochemistry tests which require heparinized plasma or whole blood for analysis.
  - *Additive:* Sodium or lithium heparin. Inhibits thrombin formation to prevent clotting
  - *Laboratory uses:* ABG analysis and osmotic fragility test.
- **Gray top tube:**
  - *Additive:* Potassium oxalate and sodium fluoride. Potassium oxalate acts as an anticoagulant and sodium fluoride acts as an antiglycolytic agent that inhibits enolase enzyme of glycolysis to ensure that no further glucose breakdown occurs within the sample after it is taken. Potassium oxalate removes calcium and acts as an anticoagulant.
  - *Laboratory uses:* Estimation of blood glucose
- **Light blue top tube**
  - *Additive:* Anticoagulant; sodium citrate. Binds and remove calcium to prevent blood from clotting
  - *Laboratory uses:* Hematology tests involving coagulation studies which include PT (Prothrombin time), TT (thrombin time) and factor assays.

- ❖ **Purple top tube:**
  - *Additive:* Anticoagulant; EDTA (Ethylenediaminetetraacetic acid). It removes calcium preventing clotting of blood
  - *Laboratory uses:* Generally used for hematology tests where whole blood is required for analysis like complete blood count, blood film for abnormal cells or malaria parasites, total leucocyte count, differential leucocyte count, platelets, Hb electrophoresis, erythrocyte sedimentation rate, HbA1C, blood bank testing (cross match, blood grouping).
- ❖ **Red top tube:**
  - *Additive:* None or contains silica particles which act as clot activators. Clot activator promotes blood clotting.
  - *Laboratory uses:* Used for biochemistry tests requiring serum, blood bank, and serology/Immunology (Hepatitis A, B, C, rheumatoid factor, HIV, viral antibodies)
- ❖ **Royal blue top tube:**
  - *Additive:* Sodium heparin and sodium EDTA. Inhibits thrombin formation to prevent clotting.
  - *Laboratory uses:* Trace elements, such as zinc, copper, lead and mercury.
- ❖ **Yellow top tube:**
  - *Additive:* anticoagulant SPS (Sodium polyanethol sulfonate) and ACD (acid citrate dextrose). Prevents the blood from clotting.
  - *Laboratory uses:* Blood and body fluid cultures (HLA, DNA, paternity).

Order of Draw

The order of draw is a special sequence of tube collection that reduces the risk of specimen contamination by microorganisms (e.g., blood cultures) and additive carry over, which affects the test results. Recommended order of draw is as given below:

- ❖ Sterile tube (e.g., blood culture)
- ❖ Coagulation tube (Blue top)
- ❖ Serum tube with/without clot activator (Red top, yellow top)
- ❖ Heparin tube (Green top)
- ❖ EDTA tube (Purple top)
- ❖ Glycolytic inhibitor tube (Gray top)

Table 4.1: Commonly used color-coded vacuum tubes, their additives and uses in laboratory.

Tube cap color	Additive	Use
Green	Anticoagulant (Lithium heparin/sodium heparin)	ABG analysis Osmotic fragility test
Grey	Potassium oxalate and sodium fluoride	Blood glucose
Light blue	Sodium citrate	**Hematology tests** involving coagulation studies which include PT (Prothrombin time), TT (Thrombin time) and factor assays
Purple	Anticoagulant; EDTA (Ethylenediaminetetraacetic acid)	**Biochemistry:** HbA1C **Hematology:** Complete blood count, blood film for abnormal cells or malaria parasites, total leukocyte count, differential leucocyte count, platelets, Hb electrophoresis, erythrocyte sedimentation rate (ESR) **Blood bank:** Cross match, blood grouping
Red	None/ or clot activator (silica particles). Clot activator promotes blood clotting	**Biochemistry** tests requiring serum, **blood bank**, and **serology**
Royal blue	Anticoagulant; Sodium heparin and sodium EDTA	Trace elements such as zinc, copper, lead and mercury
Yellow	Anticoagulant (SPS, sodium polyanethole sulfonate ACD: acid citrate dextrose)	Blood and body fluid cultures (HLA, DNA and paternity testing)

URINE SAMPLE COLLECTION

Urine is the second most common sample received in the biochemistry laboratory after the blood samples.

Types of Urine Samples and their Collection

Random Sample

* This is collected at any time of during the day. Usually used only for routine screening.
* For sample collection, the patient is given a non-sterile collection container **(Figure 4.3)** and instructed to collect a mid-stream specimen in the container. This type of specimen is routinely used for urinalysis and may not be used for a culture and sensitivity.

First Morning Sample/ First Voided Sample

* This is the first sample when the patient gets up in the morning. A first voided specimen is the most concentrated and is the preferred specimen for **microscopic examinations**. This is also the sample choice for the urine constituents to detect protein, HCG, and other substances.
* For sample collection, the patient is given a urine container to take home. Because urine is not stable, the specimen should be returned to the laboratory within one hour of collection. If that is not possible, the specimen should be refrigerated until it can be tested.

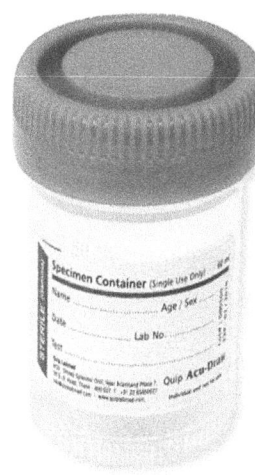

Figure 4.3: Universal urine container.

Timed Specimens

* These samples are collected at specific intervals during the day, such as 1, 4 or 24 hours. Twenty-four hour urine specimens are required for creatinine clearance tests and many other hormone studies.
* For sample collection, the patient is given a large container (1000–5000 mL capacity) containing preservative **(Figure 4.4)** that is labeled with the patient's name and date. Patient is advised to discard first morning sample on the day of collection and to collect all subsequent urine voided till next morning, including first voided sample. The 24-hour urine specimen is brought to the laboratory as soon as possible as the 24-hour period is over.

Clean-Catch Midstream Specimen

* In this case, the patient is instructed to clean the genitalia with water and soap. Then the midstream sample is collected in a universal sterile container.
* These are used for the bacteriological culture. Caution should be taken that the container should not touch the genitalia. Bring the specimen to the lab within 1 hour of collection or store refrigerated for up to 24 hours.

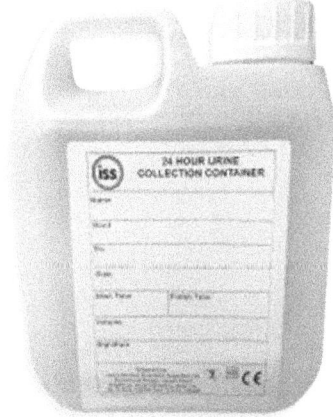

Figure 4.4: 24-hour urine collection container.

Catheterized Specimen

* These are usually collected from seriously-ill patients who are already catheterized or can insert the catheter into the urinary bladder to collect the sample who are unable to void urine. This procedure is done only by especially trained staffs.
* These are used for the microbiological examination of critically-ill patients.

Urine Storage and Preservation

The stability of some of the components excreted in the urine is affected by the change in pH that occurs in the collected sample. Urine pH often becomes more alkaline upon collection due to the presence and ongoing metabolism of bacteria and viable cells that are excreted.

- Use of preservatives reduce bacterial growth; decrease the decomposition of the chemicals associated with variable handling and storage conditions.
- Unpreserved urine specimens are subjected both to microbiologic decomposition and to inherent chemical changes.

Various urine preservatives are:
- Refrigeration of samples till analysis
- 6N HCl
- Boric acid
- Formalin (formaldehyde) is the best for urine sediments.
- Sodium fluoride
- Phenol
- Toluene
- Thymol
- Commercial preservative tablets

QUESTIONS

1. Enumerate different types of biological samples.
2. Give methods of collection of blood sample.
3. Describe color-coded vacuum evacuated tubes, their additives and uses in laboratory.
4. Describe types of urine samples.
5. Describe collection of different types of urine samples.
6. Write additives used in grey evacuated tube and its importance.
7. Enumerate different types of urine preservatives.
8. What are vacutainer tubes?
9. Mention the different vacutainer tubes and their uses.
10. What is the difference between plasma and serum?

EXPERIMENT 5

Quality Control

COMPETENCY	LEARNING OBJECTIVES
BI11.16 Observe the use of commonly used equipments/techniques in biochemistry laboratory including: pH meter, paper chromatography of amino acid, protein, electrophoresis, TLC, PAGE, electrolyte analysis by ISE, ABG analyzer, ELISA, immunodiffusion, autoanalyzer, quality control and DNA isolation from blood/tissue.	1. Describe types of errors observed in laboratory. 2. Describe terms and definitions used in clinical laboratory. 3. Describe internal and external quality control. 4. Describe interpretation of quality control data by graphical and statistical methods. 5. Describe Levey Jennings (L–J) Chart and Westgard rules.

INTRODUCTION

Quality control (QC) in a clinical laboratory plays an important role in detecting deficiencies and reducing errors in laboratory's analytical process prior to the release of patient's results. The purpose of quality control in the clinical laboratory is to ensure that the results being reported are accurate and precise.

The results of various tests provided by the laboratory are very important for the diagnosis and treatment of the disease. Even a small error could lead to serious consequences, wrong diagnosis and wrong treatment. It may be critical to the patient. This not only leads to prolonged hospitalization but also an additional financial burden on the patient. So, the results generated by the laboratory should be accurate.

TYPES OF ERRORS IN A CLINICAL LABORATORY

There are a number of potential errors which can affect the quality of the clinical laboratory results. These errors can occur in **preanalytical, analytical** and **post-analytical** phases.

Preanalytical Phase

These are the errors occur before the sample is analyzed in the laboratory. There are a number of things which can go wrong from the time when the sample is collected from the patient till it is transported to the laboratory for analysis. These errors are as follows:

- **Wrong patient information,** such as name, gender, age, ward, medical history, etc., can affect the values of analytes.
- **Improper collection of the blood sample**: The results will be affected if the sample is collected in a vacutainer other than the one which is recommended for analysis of a particular analyte for, e.g., vacutainer containing sodium citrate is used in place of sodium fluoride for analysis of plasma glucose.

- ❖ **Inadequate quantity of the sample**
- ❖ **Improper handling of the sample**: Improper handling of the sample can lead to hemolysis of the sample before it reaches the laboratory for analysis. Grossly hemolyzed sample should always be rejected as lysis of blood cells leads to release of certain intracellular chemicals and enzymes which will lead to increase in levels of potassium, phosphates and transaminases.
- ❖ **Incorrect sample storage**: If a sample has not been properly stored or a blood sample has been left overnight before being sent to the laboratory, it will become hemolyzed in 24 hours especially at a warm temperature.

Analytical Phase

The analytical phase begins from the time when the patient's specimen is prepared for analysis to the time when the test result becomes available.

- ❖ Potential analytical errors which may affect the quality of the results obtained include:
  - Sample measurement,
  - Sample pretreatment,
  - Reagent volume measurement,
  - Sample and reagent mixing,
  - Incubation, reaction timing, and
  - Calculations.
- ❖ These errors may arise in conjunction with the supplementary use of analytical equipment, such as glassware, pipettes, etc., which may not have been properly washed and calibrated.
- ❖ It is very important that the reagents should be prepared according to the instructions given by the manufacturer and also the reagents should be properly stored when not in use.
- ❖ Commonly, the analytical errors are seen after the use of expired reagents and controls and calibrators, blockade in aspiration system of reagents and samples.
- ❖ During the analytical phase, the quality of the laboratory can be maintained by running internal quality control (IQC) daily and participating in external quality assessment (EQA).

Post-Analytical Phase

Post-analytical phase mainly deals with the reporting of results after the completion of analytical phase in a timely manner and in an accepted format that can be understood and correctly interpreted by healthcare professionals. The most common post-analytical errors include the reports being not legible and also delay in delivering the reports to the clinician or the patients.

TERMS AND DEFINITIONS USED IN CLINICAL LABORATORY

Analytical errors influence the **accuracy, precision, sensitivity, specificity** and **reproducibility** and **repeatability** of the analytical methods.

- ❖ **Accuracy**: Accuracy refers to the closeness of the measured value of an analyte to its 'true' value in the given sample. Closer the measurement to the actual value, greater will be the accuracy.
- ❖ **Precision**: Precision refers to the reproducibility (consistency) of the test. The extent of variation of results obtained for the same analyte on the same sample by repeated determinations is precision. A test is said to be precise, if its repeated estimated values on the same sample are close to each other. It reflects the correctness of procedure. Precision is quantitatively expressed as Standard Deviation (SD) or more precisely as Coefficient of Variation (CV) of the results in a set of replicate measurements. Hence, good precision means least CV. Accuracy and precision can be understood with help of the **'dart board'** analogy where the center of the target corresponds with highest accuracy and precision **(Figures 5.1A to C)**.
- ❖ **Specificity** describes to the ability of a method to measure exclusively the component of interest. A lack of specificity could lead to a falsely elevated result where the test is measuring components other than the analyte of interest.

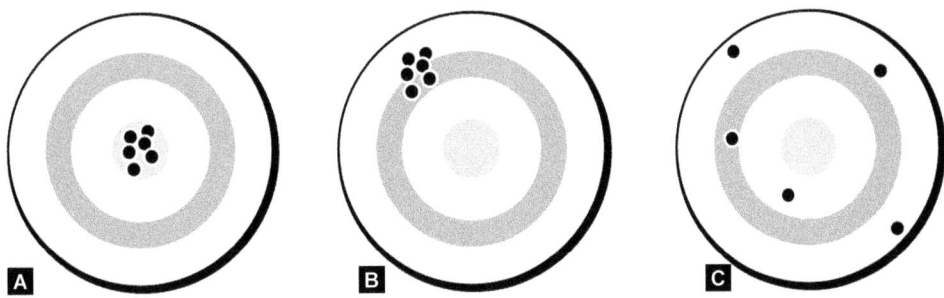

Figures 5.1A to C: Accuracy and precision: : (A) Precise and accurate; (B) Inaccurate but precise; (C) Inaccurate and imprecise.

For example, blood glucose can be estimated both by reduction (chemical) method and enzymatic method. Reduction method is nonspecific, in the sense, chemical reagent reacts with many other reducing substances found in the blood along with glucose giving higher value than the actual. Enzymatic methods are specific; enzyme reacts only with glucose to give true value of glucose.
- **Sensitivity** is the ability of a method to estimate even the minute quantities of the component of biological sample. It will subsequently affect both precision and accuracy.

INTERNAL AND EXTERNAL QUALITY CONTROL

Analytical errors must be detected at an early stage in order to minimize them. The strategy for their detection consists of specific quality control methods which are divided in two categories:
1. **Internal quality control (IQC):** Internal quality control is performed daily in the laboratory using controls whose values are known. The main purpose of IQC is to check the precision (reproducibility) of the method.
2. **External quality control (EQC):** External quality control includes the participation of the laboratory in an **external quality assessment scheme** (EQAS) which provides samples for analysis every month. They have to be analyzed by the laboratory professionals using the same procedures as used for testing of quality control samples and patient samples. The results obtained from analysis of EQC samples are reported to the external quality assessment scheme (EQAS). They then provide a report for the participating laboratory based on mean, coefficient of variation (CV) and standard deviation index of the all the participating laboratories.

INTERPRETATION OF QUALITY CONTROL DATA

The interpretation of quality control data is done with the help of both **graphical** and **statistical methods**. Quality control data is most commonly visualized with the help of quality control (QC) charts which include **Levey-Jennings (LJ) Charts** and **Westgard rules.**

Statistical Methods Used in Laboratory for Quality Control

Statistical method can be described by their **mean/average, standard deviation, coefficient of variation (CV)** and **standard deviation index**
- **Mean:** It is the most commonly used term. Mean is defined as the arithmetic average of a group of values and is determined by summing the values and dividing by the number of values.
- **Standard deviation (SD or s)** is the measure of the degree of deviation of a value from the mean and is used to assess **precision**. If a specimen is analyzed several times, the result would be around the mean value. The mean difference of each value from the mean is SD.
- **Coefficient of variation (CV):** The coefficient of variation (CV) is defined as the ratio of standard deviation to the mean and is expressed as percentage. It is another measure of percentage of **inaccuracy.** A CV of 3% is regarded as ideal result while 5% is acceptable. Values higher than 5% are wrong.

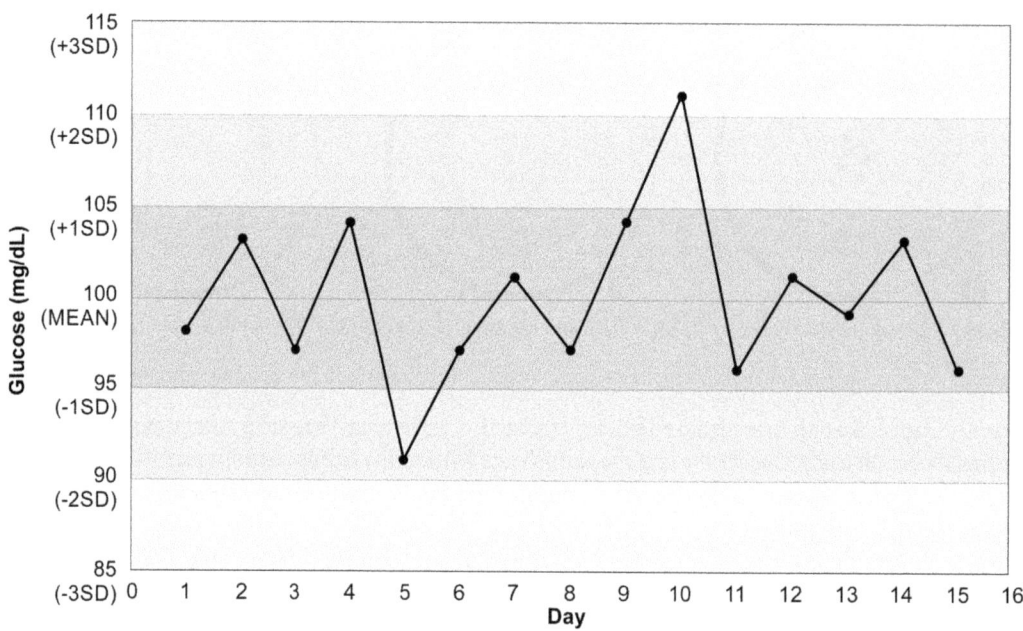

Figure 5.2: Levey Jennings plot for measurements of internal quality control of blood glucose.
[Day-wise glucose values (mg/dL) in control samples plotted (85–115). The patient glucose report is reported only if control values on L–J plot for that day are within ±1SD]

LEVEY JENNINGS (L–J) CHART AND WESTGARD RULES

The use of Levey Jennings chart (L-J chart) is one of the most commonly used charts to monitor quality control results. It is a graphical method. The dates of analyzes are plotted along the X-axis and control values are plotted along the Y-axis. The value of controls as mean ±1SD, mean ±2SD and mean ±3SD are also indicated on the Y-axis. The deviation of the results from the mean especially, when the results are greater mean ±2SD from the mean, indicate the rejection of run. An example of L-J chart is shown in **Figure 5.2** for quality control of glucose.

Reading the Chart

- If the analysis is satisfactory the points that are plotted will be scattered evenly on either side of midline within ± 1SD limit. This pattern shows that accuracy is maintained.
- Values falling within ± 2SD limit are acceptable while values at ± 2SD limit and above are warning limit, i.e., reanalysis of the control is required.
- Values at ± 3SD limit are action limit. When six consecutive values fall above or below the mean line it shows that the assay is out of control.
- In case, the value is above or below + 2SD, it indicates that the reagent or standard is deteriorated. The assay should be repeated with fresh reagents and standard (Sometimes the control serum itself deteriorates due to improper storage. Fresh control serum is to be replaced).

Westgard Rules

The rules were originally developed by **James Westgard**. The rules are applied to the Levey–Jennings chart. It also helps in deciding whether the analytical run is in control or out of control. Shorthand notations are used to abbreviate different control rules, such as 1–2s to indicate 1 control measurement exceeding 2s control limits. These are defined as follows:
- **Rule 1–2s**: It indicates one control result has exceeded the established mean ± 2SD range. This is a "warning rule," which does not indicate an "out-of-control" condition, but is intended to initiate further testing.
- **Rule 1–3s**: It indicates one control result has exceeded the established mean ± 3SD range. This is a "rejection rule," which is sensitive to random error.

EXPERIMENT 5: Quality Control

- ❖ **Rule 2-2s**: It indicates that two consecutive control results have exceeded the same mean ± 2SD limit. This is a "rejection rule".
- ❖ **Rule 4S**: It indicates that one control value exceeds the mean by +2SD and the other control value exceeds the mean by −2SD. The range between the two results will therefore exceed 4SD. This is a "rejection rule", hence, the run is rejected.
- ❖ **Rule 4-1s**: It indicates four consecutive control results have exceeded the same mean ± 1SD limit. This may indicate the need to perform instrument maintenance or reagent calibration. This is a "rejection rule".
- ❖ **Rule 10-x**: It indicates ten consecutive control results have fallen on the same side of the mean or target value. So the run has to be rejected. This is a "rejection rule".

QUESTIONS

1. **Using blood urea values of five days:**
   a. Calculate the mean and plot a Levy–Jennings graph from the given blood urea values.
   b. Comment whether 50 mg/dL of blood urea is within the acceptable range or not by plotting on graph.
   c. Which Westgard's rule is obeyed in the above case?

Day	1	2	3	4	5
Blood urea (mg/dL)	34	28	36	29	33

- The + 1 SD values for blood urea is + 3 mg/dL
- The + 2 SD values for blood urea is + 6 mg/dL
- The + 3 SD values for blood urea is + 9 mg/dL

2. **Using cholesterol values of five days:**
   a. Calculate the mean and plot a Levy–Jennings graph from the given cholesterol values.
   b. Comment whether 220 mg/dL of blood cholesterol is within the acceptable range or not by plotting on graph.
   c. Which Westgard's rule is obeyed in the above case?

Day	1	2	3	4	5
Blood cholesterol (mg/dL)	154	162	156	175	153

- The + 1 SD values for cholesterol is + 8 mg/dL
- The + 2 SD values for cholesterol is + 16 mg/dL
- The + 3 SD values for cholesterol is + 24 mg/dL

EXPERIMENT 6

pH Meter and Preparation of Buffers

COMPETENCY	LEARNING OBJECTIVES
BI11.2 Describe the preparation of buffers and estimation of pH.	1. Describe principle of pH meter, measurement of pH and its applications.
BI11.16 Observe the use of commonly used equipments/ techniques in biochemistry laboratory including: pH meter, paper chromatography of amino acid, protein electrophoresis, TLC, PAGE, electrolyte analysis by ISE, ABG analyzer, ELISA, immunodiffusion, autoanalyzer, quality control and DNA isolation from blood/tissue.	2. Describe buffer and its importance.
	3. Demonstrate preparation of phosphate buffer in laboratory and measurement of pH of buffer using a pH meter.
BI11.19 Outline the basic principles involved in the functioning of instruments commonly used in a biochemistry laboratory and their applications.	

INTRODUCTION

A pH meter is a scientific instrument used to measure the pH value of a given water-based solution **(Figure 6.1)**. A pH meter is basically a voltmeter able to detect very low voltages. An amplifier magnifies this electric potential, and the voltmeter reads out that value and shows it on the scale. The scale is so calibrated that we can interpret this voltage reading as pH values. The pH value of a solution is basically the strength of the hydrogen ions in it.

The pH of the solution is measured by two ways; by using a pH strip or pH indicator and a pH meter. An approximate idea of the pH of by using a solution can be obtained using indicators. The most convenient and reliable method for measuring pH is by the use of a pH meter.

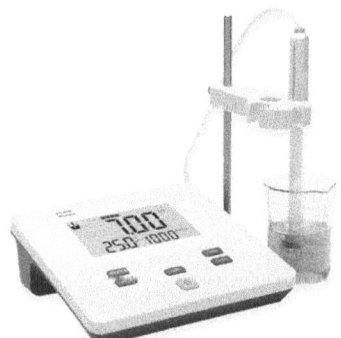

Figure 6.1: pH meter.

PRINCIPLE OF pH METER, MEASUREMENT OF pH AND ITS APPLICATIONS

Principle

A pH meter measures electric potential (electric current) using two electrodes inserted into the liquid to create an electrical circuit. One of these electrodes, called the **reference standard electrode** and the other electrode, known as the **glass electrode.**

- The **glass electrode** consists of very thin glass bulb which is sensitive to hydrogen ion concentration of test sample solution. Glass bulb is filled with 0.1M HCl connected to a platinum wire via Ag-AgCl electrode. A potential is developed across the thin glass of the bulb which depends on the pH of the solution in which it is immersed. The glass electrode in the test solution constitutes a half cell and the measuring circuit is completed by a **reference electrode** which is not sensitive to hydrogen ions.
- The **reference electrode** is standard and has constant potential. The reference electrode does not respond to test sample solution. The reference electrode commonly used is the **calomel electrode**. It consists of glass tube which is filled with **saturated solution of KCl** and porous KCl crystals are plugged at the tip. In this solution, mercury electrode is dipped, the tip of which has porous plug of **mercury calomel paste (Figure 6.2)**.
- The pH meter measures the potential difference between both glass and reference electrodes. The potential difference is used to measure the hydrogen ion concentration indicating the pH of given solution. The calculated difference in electrical potential relates to the hydrogen ion concentration indicating the pH of given solution.

Modern pH meters use a single combined electrode in which glass and reference electrode are placed into a rod like structure.

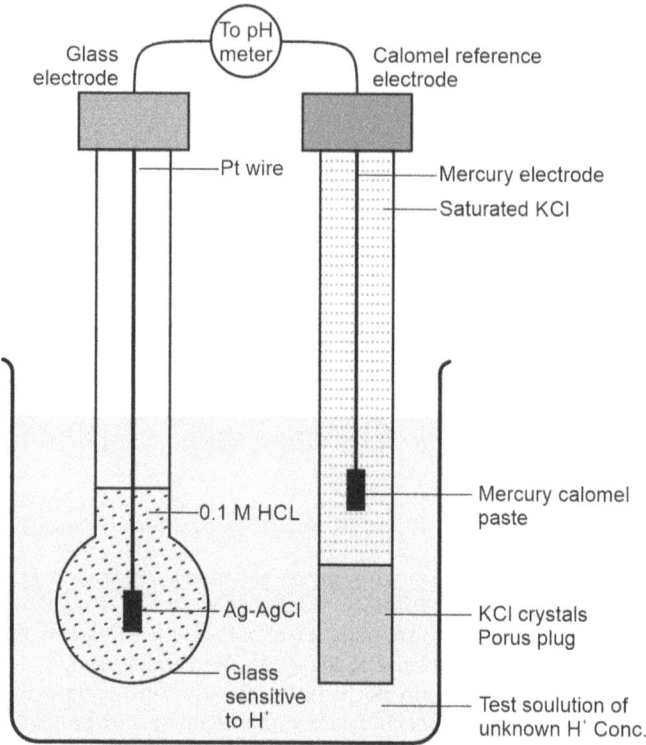

Figure 6.2: Electrode system for the measurement of pH.

Measurement of pH

The electrodes or probes are inserted into the solution to be tested. On immersion in the solution to be tested, the H^+ ion in the test solution moves close to the external side of glass bulb. The H^+ ions present inside the bulb also moves close to glass membrane (internal side of the bulb). This causes the difference in the concentration of hydrogen ion across the glass membrane causing difference in the potential (voltage) across the bulb. The electronic amplifier detects the difference in electrical potential between two electrodes generated in the measurement and converts the potential difference to pH units.
- When the hydrogen ion concentration inside the glass bulb is less than the outside solution (test solution), then the given solution is acidic and hence the pH is lower than 7.
- When the hydrogen ions concentration across the membrane is same then it is called as neutral pH and the pH is equal to 7.
- If the concentration of hydrogen ion of inside the bulb is more than outside solution then the given solution is alkaline and the pH is more than 7.

Application of pH Meter

pH meters are widely used in a variety of applications where the pH of a solution needs to be measured, including:
- **Clinical laboratories:** To measure pH of various biological fluids, to adjust pH of buffer solution which are used in enzyme assays and to adjust pH of various reagents used in biochemical assays.
- **Scientific research:** To measure the pH of chemical solutions and other materials.
- **Water treatment:** To monitor the pH of drinking water, and wastewater.
- **Industrial manufacturing:** To monitor the pH of chemicals, liquids, and other materials.

- **Food processing:** To measure the pH of foods and beverages. This is important for ensuring that the pH of the products is within a safe and acceptable range, and to ensure that they have the desired taste and texture.
- **Agricultural applications:** To measure the pH of soil and water in order to optimize crop growth and productivity.

BUFFER: DEFINITION AND ITS IMPORTANCE

Definition
Buffers are solutions that resist changes in pH when small amounts of acid or base are added. Buffer solutions are composed of a mixture of weak acid (the proton donor; HA) and a salt of its conjugate base (the proton acceptor; A⁻).

Commonly Used Laboratory Buffers
- Acetate buffer (Acetic acid-sodium acetate)
- Bicarbonate buffer (H_2CO_3/$NaHCO_3$)
- Phosphate buffer (H_2PO_4/ Na_2HPO_4)
- Barbitone (veronal) buffer (sodium diethyl barbiturate/hydrochloric acid)
- Citrate buffer (citrate acid/sodium citrate)
- Tris buffer (tris amino methane and hydrochloric acid)

Mechanism of Buffer
- Buffers resist the change in pH because they contain an acidic component; HA to neutralize OH⁻ ions, and a basic component; A⁻ to neutralize H⁺ ions
- When a strong acid is added to a buffer solution, the H⁺ ions donated by the acid are accepted and neutralized by the base member (A⁻) of the buffer. In contrast, when strong base is added to a buffer solution a rise in OH⁻ ions in the solution are neutralized by an acidic component of buffer (HA).

Importance of Buffer
- Buffers are used in almost all biochemical reactions to maintain optimum pH conditions. For example in:
  - Various qualitative and quantitative estimations
  - Electrophoretic separation of proteins, lipoproteins and hemoglobin
- Almost all biological processes are pH dependent. Even a slight change in pH can result in metabolic acidosis or alkalosis, resulting in severe metabolic complications. The purpose of a buffer in a biological system is to maintain intracellular and extracellular pH within a very narrow range (7.35 to 7.45).
- The three main buffer systems in human being are **bicarbonate, phosphate** and **protein**

PREPARATION OF PHOSPHATE BUFFER SOLUTION IN LABORATORY

A phosphate buffer solution is one of the commonly used buffer solution in biological laboratories and commonly used in hematology laboratory for diluting the stains.

The phosphate buffers consist of a mixture of monobasic dihydrogen phosphate (NaH_2PO_4) and dibasic monohydrogen phosphate (Na_2HPO_4). By varying the amount of each salt, a range of buffers can be prepared **(Table 6.1)**

Materials Required for the Preparation of Phosphate Buffer Solution (pH 5.8 to 7.4)
- **0.2 M NaH_2PO_4 (monosodium phosphate):** 4.6 g of NaH_2PO_4/1000 mL water
- **0.2 M Na_2HPO_4 (disodium phosphate):** 35.61 g of Na_2HPO_4/1000 mL water
- Phosphoric acid (to make the pH more acidic as per the case)
- Sodium hydroxide (to make the pH more alkaline as per the case)
- pH meter

Procedure

Mix monosodium phosphate and disodium phosphate solution to get required pH as shown in the **Table 6.1.** Measure the pH of each buffer solution by **pH meter** and adjust the pH with adding acid or base. If the mixed solution shows pH more than the required pH, use phosphoric acid to decrease the pH, if it is less than the required one, then add base, sodium hydroxide to increase the pH.

Table 6.1: Preparation of phosphate buffer of different pH values.

pH	mL of 0.2M NaH_2PO_4	mL of 0.2M Na_2HPO_4
6.9	44.6	55.4
7.0	38.8	61.2
7.2	28.0	72.0
7.4	19.0	81.0

QUESTIONS

1. Write applications of pH meter.
2. Write principle of pH meter.
3. Define buffer, give its importance.
4. Give commonly used laboratory buffers
5. Write mechanism of buffer action.

EXPERIMENT 7

Principles of Colorimetry and Spectrophotometry

COMPETENCY	LEARNING OBJECTIVES
BI11.6 Describe the principles of colorimetry. **BI11.18** Discuss the principles of spectrophotometry. **BI11.19** Outline the basic principles involved in the functioning of instruments commonly used in biochemistry laboratory and their applications.	1. Demonstrate principle, components, functioning and applications of colorimetry. 2. Demonstrate principle, components, technique and applications of spectrophotometry.

INTRODUCTION

The clinical chemistry laboratory is involved with quantitative estimation of various biochemical analytes in blood and body fluids. The most widely used method for determining the concentration of biochemical compounds is **colorimetry** which is based on **photometry**. Photometry is the measurement of intensity of light absorbed in the ultraviolet (UV) or visible (VIS) or infrared (IR) range. The most widely used photometric techniques for quantitative analysis in clinical chemistry are:
- Colorimetry (visible spectrum)
- Spectrophotometry (ultraviolet, visible and infrared spectrum)

The principle of photometry is based on **Beer-Lambert Law**. According to this law, when a monochromatic light passes through a solution of a certain path length, then the amount of light absorbed by the solution is directly proportional to the concentration of a substance and the path length. Mathematically, Beer-Lambert Law is expressed as:

$$A = kCL$$

Where:
- A = Absorbance,
- k = Proportionality constant or absorptivity
- C = Concentration of the analyte
- L = Light path (Path Length)

This equation forms the basis of quantitative analysis by both **colorimetry** and **spectrophotometry**.

PRINCIPLE, COMPONENTS, TECHNIQUE AND APPLICATIONS OF COLORIMETER

Principle of Colorimeter

Colorimetry is an analytical technique used to determine the concentration of substances (analytes) in a sample by measuring the amount of **light absorbed** (absorbance) when a monochromatic light of specific wavelength is passed through the sample. The amount of light absorbed by the solution is directly proportional to the concentration of a substance as described by Beer-Lambert law.

Relationship between Absorption and Transmittance

When light passes through colored solution, some amount of light is absorbed by the solution, depending on the concentration of the light absorbing compound, while remaining light is transmitted. The amount of light absorbed is termed as "**Absorbance**" (A) or "**Optical density**" (OD), whereas the amount of light transmitted is termed as "**Transmittance**" (T).

Components of Colorimeter

The main components of a colorimeter are (**Figures 7.1A and B**):

- **A lamp (light source):** A lamp provides light in visible region of the spectrum. Usually, tungsten lamp is the source of light.
- **Adjustable slit:** The light emerging from tungsten lamp is allowed to pass through a narrow adjustable slit.
- **Condensing lens:** Provides parallel beam of light.
- **Filter:** Filter provides the desired monochromatic light (of single wavelength) by filtering other wavelengths. The color of the filter is complementary to the color of the solution (**Table 7.1**). This allows only appropriate wavelength of light to pass through the colored solution.
- **Cuvette (sample holder):** A special glass tube, which holds the solution to be analyzed in a colorimeter, is called cuvette. Cuvette should have uniform thickness, inner diameter and refractive index. Corvettes usually have ond cm light path.
- **Photo detector:** Produces a current in response to the light impinging upon it.
- **Galvanometer readout device:** That measures electric current generated by the photocell to optical density or % transmittance.

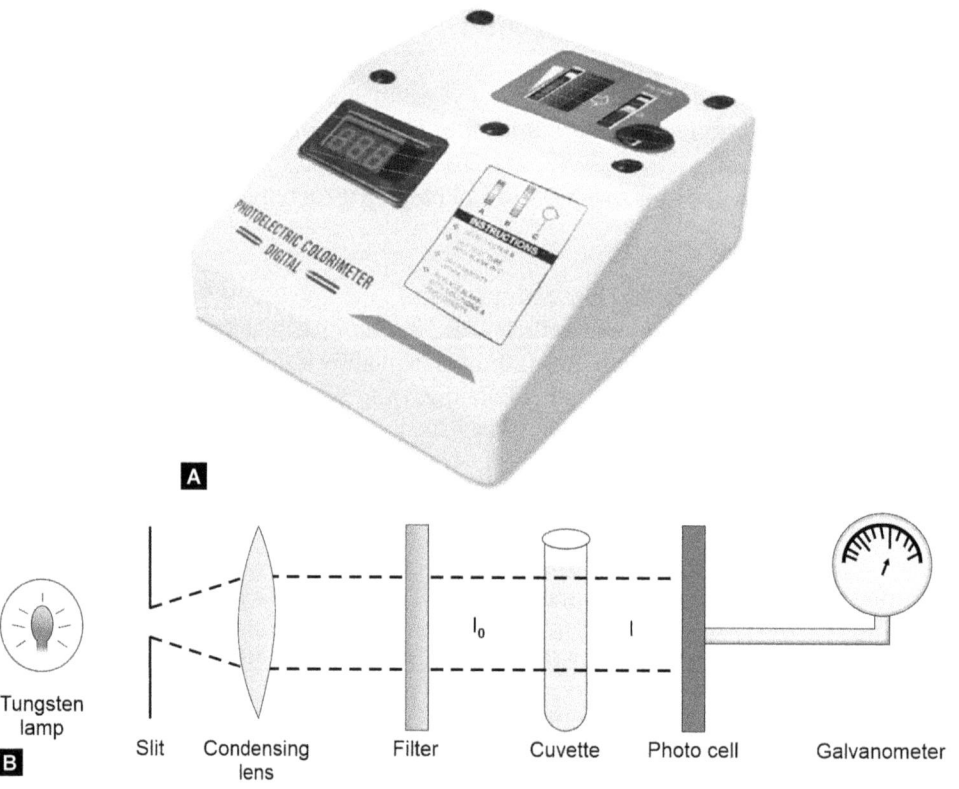

Figures 7.1A and B: Colorimeter and its components.

Table 7.1: Complementary colors for selection of filters.

Filter	Color of solution
Blue	Red
Purple	Green
Yellow	Violet
Orange	Blue green

Functioning of the Colorimeter

Preparation of Solution for Investigation

In colorimetric estimation, it is necessary to prepare three solutions:
1. Blank (B)
2. Standard (S)
3. Test (T)

Blank: Since some colors comes from the reagents used in the procedure, which is in addition to the color produced by the substance, which is desired to be estimated. To eliminate the effect of light absorption by the reagents used, a **blank** is also run by similarly treating at the same time a same volume of distilled water. Two types of blank are used:
- **Water blank:** It is used to adjust the OD to zero and % T to 100.
- **Reagent blank:** It is prepared by adding all reagents except the substance to be estimated.

Standard solution: It is a solution of known concentration of the substance in pure form to be estimated. Both concentration and OD of the standard solution are known, therefore the concentration of unknown can be calculated.

Test solution or unknown: The test solution is made by treating a specific volume of the test sample with reagents as mention in the procedure.

Steps in the Operation of the Colorimeter

- Place glass filter recommended in the procedure in the filter slot.
- Fill the cuvette to about 3/4th with the distilled water and place in the cuvette slot.
- Switch 'on' the instrument and allow it to warm-up 4 to 5 minutes.
- Press the button adjusts the **'coarse'** and **'fine'** knobs to give zero optical activity in the galvanometer. Release the button.
- Take blank solution in an identical cuvette and placed it in the cuvette slot, press the button and read the optical density (OD), without disturbing the previous adjusted **'coarse'** and **fine** knobs. Release the button. Let the OD be **'B'.**
- Transfer the **'blank'** solution as completely as possible to the original test tube.
- Next take **'test'** solution in the same cuvette and as with **'blank'** read the OD. Let it be **'T'**.
- Transfer the test solution back to the original test tube.
- Finally take **'standard'** solution in the same cuvette and as before record the OD. Let it be **'S'**.
- Transfer the **'standard'** solution back to the original test tube, wash the cuvette. Satisfactory results are obtained only when the OD values are in the range 0.1 to 0.7.
- Put all required values in the formula given below for estimation of concentration of 'test' sample and calculate it.

Calculation of Concentration of Unknown Analyte

$$\text{Concentration of the substance in the sample (mg/dL)} = \frac{\text{OD test solution}}{\text{OD of standard}} \times \frac{\text{Conc. of standard}}{\text{Volume of sample}} \times 100$$

$$= \frac{\text{OD T} - \text{OD B}}{\text{OD S} - \text{OD B}} \times \frac{\text{Conc. of standard}}{\text{Volume of sample}} \times 100$$

Where, ODT, ODS, and ODB represents optical density of test, standard, and blank solutions respectively.

Applications of Colorimeter

❖ Colorimeter is widely used in hospital and clinical laboratory for the estimation of various biochemical parameters in various biological samples, such as blood, plasma, serum, cerebrospinal fluid (CSF), urine and other body fluids.
❖ The biochemical parameters, such as glucose, urea, creatinine, uric acid, bilirubin, lipids, total proteins, and enzymes, such as alanine aminotransferase (ALT), aspartate aminotransferase (AST), alkaline phosphatase (ALP), etc., in blood and body fluids, such as CSF, urine, pleural fluid, etc., for diagnosis of various diseases.

PRINCIPLE, COMPONENTS, TECHNIQUE AND APPLICATIONS OF SPECTROPHOTOMETRY

A Spectrophotometer is a sophisticated type of colorimeter. Both colorimetry and spectrophotometry are two analytical techniques used to determine the content of a substance in a given sample by measuring light absorption through that sample.

Difference between Colorimeter and Spectrophotometer

❖ The key difference between colorimetry and spectrophotometry is that colorimetry uses wavelengths that are only in the visible range while spectrophotometry can use wavelengths in a wider range (UV and IR also).
❖ Spectrophotometer differs from colorimeter in the type of monochromator used. Colorimeters use filter whereas spectrophotometer use prism or diffraction grating to get entire spectrum of wavelengths from which any desired wavelength of light can be selected.
❖ The main difference between colorimeter and spectrophotometer is that, colorimeter measures the **absorbance of light** whereas spectrophotometer measures the **transmittance** (reflectance) of the sample.
❖ Spectrophotometer is more expensive than filter photometer.
❖ Spectrophotometer has advantage over filter photometer of having a greater convenience and flexibility in the choice of wavelength not only in visible part of the light but also in ultraviolet and infrared region of light.

Principle of Spectrophotometry

Principle of spectrophotometer is fundamentally same as that of colorimetry, i.e., based on Beer-Lambert law as has been discussed in detail in the colorimetry.

Components of Spectrophotometer

The main components of a spectrophotometer are shown in **Figure 7.2**.
❖ **Light sources:** Types of light sources used in spectrophotometers include incandescent lamps, xenon discharge lamps, laser and light-emitting diodes (LEDs).
❖ **Entrance slit:** The incident light from light source is allowed to pass through a slit which may be inserted before the monochromatic device to convert it in beam of light.
❖ **Monochromator:** The monochromator used in spectrophotometer is prism or diffraction grating.
❖ **Cuvette:** A cuvette is a small vessel used to hold a liquid sample to be analyzed in the light path of a spectrophotometer. Cuvette should have uniform thickness, inner diameter and refractive index. Most cuvette have 1.0 cm light path.
❖ **Photo detector:** A photo detector is a device that converts light into an electric signal that is proportional to the number of photons striking its photosensitive surface. The photomultiplier tube is a commonly used photo detector in a spectrophotometer for measuring light intensity in the UV and visible regions of the spectrum.

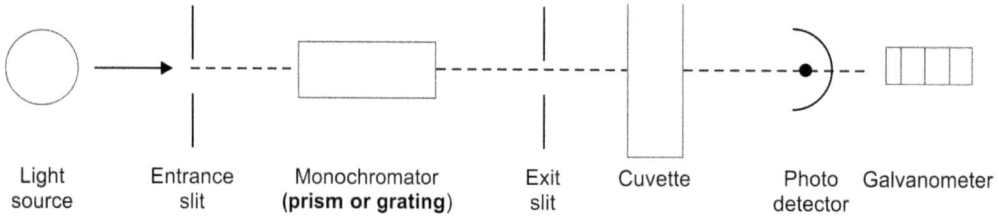

Figure 7.2: Components of spectrophotometer.

❖ **Galvanometer:** Electrical energy from a detector is displayed on some type of meter or readout system. Presently, we have digital readout devices that provide a visual numeric display of absorbance or converted values of concentrations.

Applications of Spectrophotometer

Spectrophotometers are widely used in various disciplines, such as physics, molecular biology, chemistry and biochemistry.
- ❖ It is used to determine the concentration of an analyte present in a sample.
- ❖ Spectrophotometry is an important technique used in DNA, RNA and protein isolation.
- ❖ It is one of the best methods for determination of impurities in an organic molecule.
- ❖ It can be used to determined molecular weight of a compound.
- ❖ It can be used to study kinetics of a reaction.

QUESTIONS

1. Write the principle of colorimetry.
2. Write the application of colorimetry.
3. Write the components of colorimeter.
4. What do you understand by standard solution? What is the importance of a 'blank'?
5. What is the transmittance and absorbance? How are they related?
6. What is the equation for derivation of concentration of unknown sample?
7. What is Beers-Lambert's law?
8. Write the application of spectrophotometer?
9. Write the components of spectrophotometer?
10. What are the advantages of spectrophotometer over colorimeter?
11. What are monochromatic devices used on colorimeter and spectrophotometer?
12. What are the differences between colorimeter and spectrophotometer?

EXPERIMENT 8

Electrolyte Analysis by Ion Selective Electrode

COMPETENCY	LEARNING OBJECTIVES
BI11.16 Observe the use of commonly used equipments/techniques in biochemistry laboratory including: pH meter, paper chromatography, protein electrophoresis, TLC, page, electrolyte analysis by ISE, ABG analyzer, ELISA, immunodiffusion, Autoanalyzer, quality control and DNA isolation from blood tissue.	1. Describe principle components and clinical application of ion selective electrode (ISE).

INTRODUCTION

Ion selective electrode is a widely used analytical tool for detecting **ions** in various samples of clinical, industrial, environmental, and laboratory research. Ion selective electrodes are the electrode that generates an electrical potential in the response to the specific ion present in a solution. ISEs are used in clinical chemistry for measuring ionic concentrations of various analytes, such as sodium, potassium, calcium, lithium, etc.

PRINCIPLE

It is based on the principle of potentiometry like pH meter. It contains a **reference electrode, ion-selective electrode (ISE),** and **voltmeter.** ISE consists of a **thin membrane** across which only the specific ion can be transported. The transport of ions from high concentration to low concentration through the **selective membrane** creates a potential difference which is measured with respect to a standard reference electrode (having a constant electrode potential) by voltmeter.

COMPONENTS OF ISE (FIGURE 8.1)

- **Reference electrode:** The electrode with a constant voltage made of $Ag/AgCl_2$.
- **Ion selective electrode:** That generates an electrical potential in the response to the specific ion present in a solution.
- **Voltage source:** To measure the electrode potential, a constant voltage source is needed as a reference potential.
- **Sample chamber:** Contains specimen to be measured.

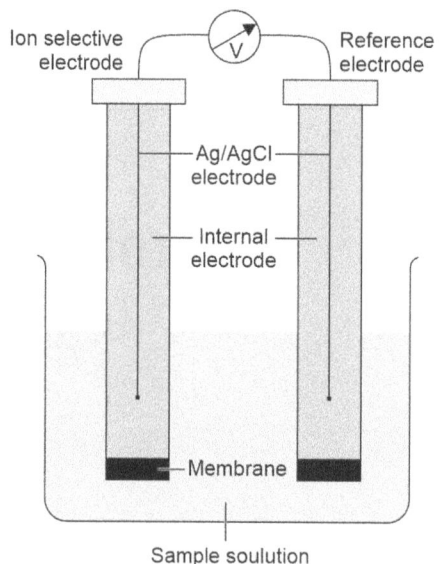

Figure 8.1: Components of ion selective electrode.

Ion Selective Electrode Types

The essential part of an ISE is the **ion-selective membrane** which is commonly placed between the sample and inner solutions that contain an analyte ion. The membrane used in ISE may be a glass, a crystalline solid, or a liquid. On the basis of nature of membrane materials, ion selective electrodes can be classified into the following major types:
1. Glass membrane electrode
2. Crystalline or solid state membrane electrodes
3. Liquid membrane electrode or Ion exchange electrodes
4. Gas sensing electrode

- **Glass membrane electrodes**: The most famous glass electrode determines H^+ activity or pH. The membrane is composed of a silicate glass. Glass electrodes can also be constructed that are sensitive to other cations, such as **sodium**.
- **Crystalline/solid state membrane electrodes**: These membranes are made from insoluble ionic conducting inorganic salts. One of the common examples of such electrodes is the **fluoride ion selective electrode.** Crystal LaF_3 (Lanthanum trifluoride) is widely used to determine F^-.
- **Liquid membrane electrode**: It contains ion-exchanger or ionophore incorporated in an inert organic liquid membrane. These are used in electrodes to measure ions such as **Potassium, Calcium**, and **Nitrate.**
- **Gas sensing electrodes:** These electrodes are used to measure dissolved gas, such as carbon dioxide, ammonia, sulfur dioxide, etc. Gas sensing electrodes have gas permeable membranes.

Applications of Ion Selective Electrode

Ion selective electrodes can be used:
- To determine various ions in aqueous solutions.
- To measure the pH of the solution.
- To monitor pollutants in natural water and effluents by measuring CN^-, F^-, S^-, Cl^-, NO_3^-, etc.
- To measure different types of ions present in the soil.

- To measure NO_3^-, NO_2^- ions in meat preservatives, and salt content in meat, fish, and fruit juices.
- To determine fluoride ions in drinking water and other drinks.
- To determine ions, such as Ca^{++}, K^+, Cl^-, etc, in body fluids, such as plasma, serum, and sweat.
- As a chemical sensor for research purposes.

QUESTIONS

1. What is ion selective electrode?
2. What is the principle of ion selective electrode?
3. What are the components of ion selective electrode?
4. Write types of ion selective electrodes.
5. Write applications ion selective electrodes.

EXPERIMENT 9

Enzyme-linked Immunosorbent Assay

COMPETENCY	LEARNING OBJECTIVES
BI11.16 Observe the use of commonly used equipments/techniques in biochemistry laboratory including: pH meter, paper chromatography, protein electrophoresis, TLC, page, electrolyte analysis by ISE, ABG analyzer, ELISA, immunodiffusion, Autoanalyzer, quality control and DNA isolation from blood tissue.	1. Describe principle, types, data interpretation and clinical application of ELISA.

INTRODUCTION

The enzyme-linked immunosorbent assay (ELISA) is an immunological assay commonly used to measure **antibodies, antigens, proteins** and **glycoproteins** and **hormones** in biological samples. These assays involve the use of catalytic properties of **enzymes** and **immunosorbent** (an absorbing material) that specifically absorbs the antigen or antibody present in serum.

PRINCIPLE OF ELISA

ELISA test is based on **antigen-antibody** reaction. ELISAs are typically performed in **microtiter plates** having number of **microwells (Figure 9.1)**. The surface of wells is coated either with **antigen** or **antibody** which is immobilized.

❖ The antigen-antibody reaction is initiated by incubating serum in a well. Antibodies or antigens present in serum are captured by corresponding antigen or antibody coated on to the solid surface. Antigen is captured if antibodies are bound to the plate and antibodies are captured if antigens are bound to the plate.

❖ After some time, the plate is washed to remove serum and unbound antibodies or antigens with a series of wash buffer.

❖ To detect the bound antibodies or antigens, **secondary antibodies** that are attached to an **enzyme,** such as **peroxidase** or **alkaline phosphatase** are added to each well.

❖ After an incubation period, the unbound secondary antibodies are washed off.

❖ Then a suitable substrate specific to the enzyme is added. Enzyme which is linked with an antibody acts on substrate and catalyzes the formation of colored product from colorless substrate.

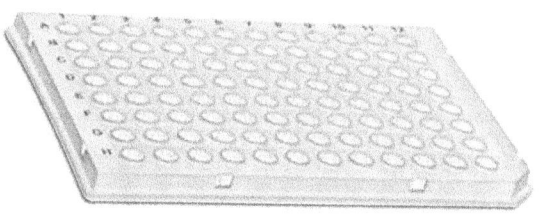

Figure 9.1: Microtiter plate.

❖ The color produced by catalytic activity of an enzyme is detected by reading the intensity of the color by colorimetrically. The intensity of the color depends on the amount of antigen or antibody in the serum.

TYPES OF ELISA

ELISA tests can be classified into four types which differ from each other in their principles.
1. Direct ELISA
2. Indirect ELISA
3. Sandwich ELISA
4. Competitive ELISA

Direct ELISA

It is used for detection of antigen in test serum. In direct ELISA, only primary antibody (targeted against the serum antigen) labeled with an enzyme is used, secondary antibodies are not needed **(Figure 9. 2)**

❖ In direct ELISA wells of microtiter plate are empty, not pre-coated with antigen or antibody. A solution of non-reacting protein, such as bovine serum albumin or casein, is added to each well in order to cover any plastic surface in the well.
❖ Test serum (containing antigen) is added into the wells. Antigen becomes attached to the solid phase by passive adsorption.
❖ After washing, the enzyme-linked primary antibodies are added which "directly" binds to the test antigen that is bound to the surface of the microtiter plate wells.
❖ After washing, a substrate for this enzyme is then added. The enzyme linked to the primary antibody reacts with the substrate to produce a color, and its intensity can be measured by ELISA reader.
❖ Intensity of the color is directly proportional to the concentration of the antigen present in the serum.

Indirect ELISA

The indirect ELISA is used for the quantitative estimation of antibodies or less commonly antigen in serum. In indirect ELISA, both a primary antibody and a secondary antibody are used. But in this case, the primary antibody is not linked (labeled) with an enzyme. Instead, the secondary antibody is labeled with an enzyme **(Figure 9. 3)**. The test is extensively used for determination of serum antibodies for diagnosis of **human immunodeficiency virus (HIV)** infection, **dengue** and many other viral infections.

❖ In this method, specimens (serum) are added to **microtiter plate wells** coated with **antigen**.
❖ Test sample containing antibody (primary) specific to antigen is added to the well.

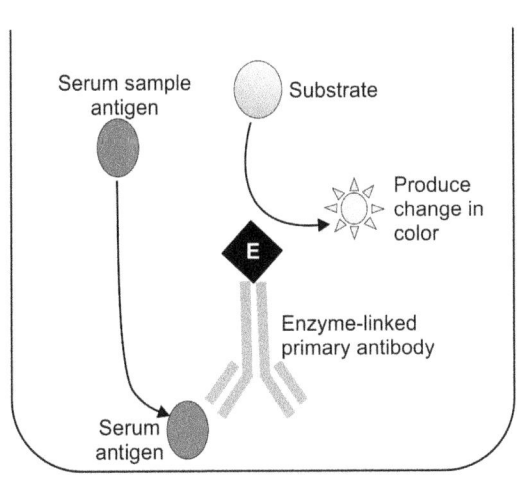

Figure 9.2: Direct ELISA.

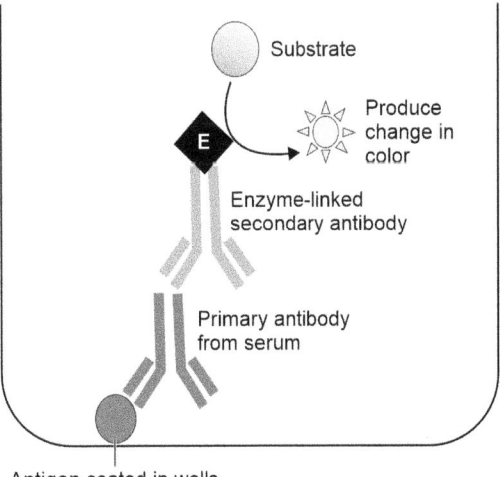

Figure 9.3: Indirect ELISA.

❖ The primary antibody present in the sample bind specifically to the antigen. After a period of incubation, the wells are washed to remove unbound antibodies.
❖ Next, secondary antibodies linked with an enzyme are added and incubated. During incubation, the **enzyme-linked secondary antibody** binds to the primary antibody.
❖ After another washing step, a **substrate** for the enzyme is added. The enzyme linked to the secondary antibody reacts with its substrate to develop a color.
❖ The concentration of primary antibody present in the serum directly correlates with the intensity of the color. The intensity of the color is measured by ELISA reader.

Sandwich ELISA

The sandwich ELISA is used for the detection of **antigen** in test serum. It is so named because the antigen gets sandwiched between a capture antibody and a detector antibody. In sandwich ELISA, it is the antibody that is coated to the plate, and this antibody is called **capture antibody** (because it captures antigen). There are two types of **sandwich ELISA: direct** and **indirect (Figures 9.4A and B)**, depending upon whether the detector antibody is a primary antibody (direct) or secondary antibody (indirect).

Direct Sandwich ELISA

❖ The microtiter well is pre-coated with the **capture antibody** specific the test antigen.
❖ The test serum (containing antigen) is added to the wells. Antigen gets attached to the capture antibody coated on the well.
❖ After washing, an **enzyme labeled primary detector antibody** specific for the antigen is added. The added **enzyme labeled primary detector antibody** binds to the antigen which is bound to capture antibody and "sandwiches" the antigen. The detector antibody can be same as the capture antibody.
❖ After washing, a substrate is added and then the enzyme reacts with substrate to produce a color that can be measured by ELISA reader.

In Indirect Sandwich ELISA

In addition to capture antibody, indirect sandwich ELISA also involves the use of unlabeled **primary antibody** and the **enzyme-linked secondary antibody (Figures 9.4A and B).** In indirect sandwich ELISA, the primary antibody is not labeled with enzyme. Another **enzyme-linked secondary antibody** is used. Thus, it is more specific than direct sandwich ELISA.
❖ Firstly, the test sample is added to the wells coated with the capture antibody and is allowed to react with the coated **capture antibodies** in the wells.

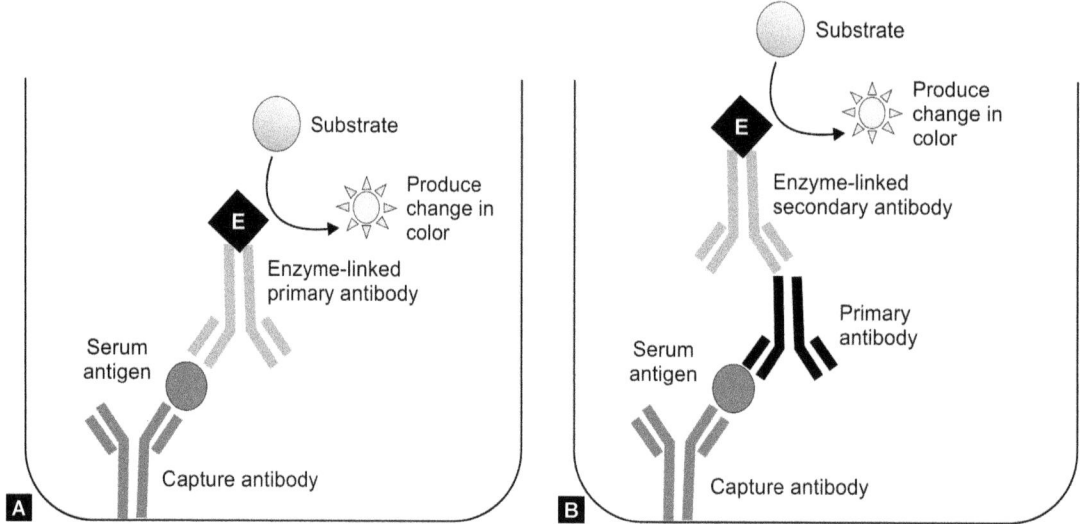

Figures 9.4A and B: Sandwich ELISA for antigen detection: (A) Direct sandwich; (B) Indirect sandwich.

- Secondly, primary antibody is added. The added **primary antibody** binds to the antigen which is bound to capture antibody and "sandwiches" the antigen.
- Thirdly, an **enzyme-linked secondary antibody** specific for the antigen is added and allowed to incubate. Enzyme-linked secondary antibody binds to primary antibody.
- After washing, the specific substrate is added. An enzyme acts on the substrate to produce a color, and its intensity can be measured by ELISA reader.

Competitive ELISA

Competitive ELISA is used for the estimation of **antigen**s or **antibodies** present in serum. Competitive ELISA is so named because, antigen in test serum competes with another antigen coated on well to bind to the primary antibody.
- Unlabeled primary antibody is first incubated in a solution with a serum which is to be analyzed for antigen.
- This antigen-antibody mixture is then added to the microtiter well which are pre-coated with the same type of antigen.
- The free antibodies present in the antigen-antibody mixture bind to the antigen coated on the well. More the test antigens present in the sample, lesser free antibodies will be available to bind to the antigens coated onto well.
- Remove free antibodies by washing. After washing enzyme-linked secondary antibody is added and incubated.
- After rewashing, a substrate is added. An enzyme acts on the substrate to produce a color, and its intensity can be measured by ELISA reader.
- Intensity of the color is **inversely proportional** to the amount of **antigen** present in the test serum.
The competitive ELISA can also be used for the detection of antibody in serum.

ELISA DATA INTERPRETATION

The ELISA assay yields three different types of data output:
- **Qualitative:** Qualitative ELISA only determines whether a particular antigen is present or not in the sample.
- **Semi-quantitative:** ELISAs can be used to compare the relative levels of antigen in assay samples, since the intensity of color will vary directly with antigen concentration
- **Quantitative:** ELISA data can be used to calculate accurately the concentrations of antigen in various samples. The concentration of the sample can be determined from the optical density value using a **standard curve.** The optical density value can be converted into concentration by use of the standard curve **(Figure 9.5)**.

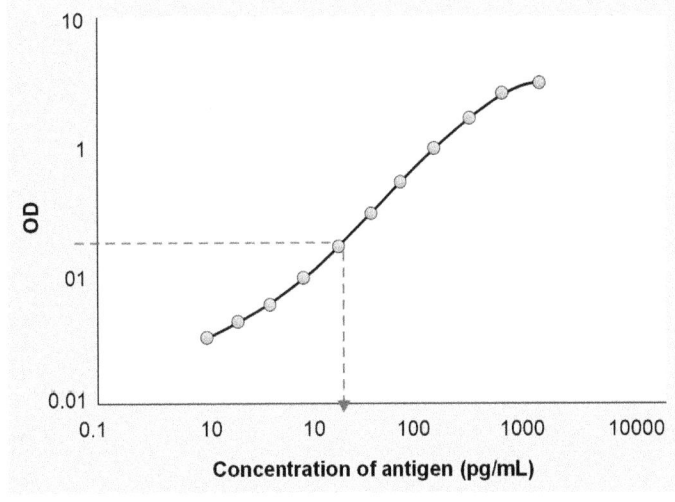

Figure 9.5: The standard calibration curve.

ELISA Standard Curve

The standard or calibration curve is used in calculating the concentration of antigen in the sample. The standard curve is derived from plotting known concentrations of a reference antigen against the optical density to produce a sigmoidal curve as shown **Figure 9.5.** The linear portion of the standard curve is used to determine, accurately the concentration of antigen present in a unknown sample. The unknown concentration can be determined directly on the graph or with curve fitting software which is typically found on ELISA plate readers.

Applications of ELISA

ELISA is extensively used in diagnosis of a wide variety of infectious as well as non-infectious diseases. Few examples of such are as follows:

SECTION A: SGD/Demo

- Detection of viral infections, such as HIV, dengue, hepatitis A and B, influenza, COVID-19, etc.
- Detection of rotavirus, *Entamoeba,* etc., in stool samples
- Detection of bacterial infections including tuberculosis, syphilis, enteric fever, etc.
- Detection of *E. coli, Campylobacter, salmonella*, etc., in food and food products.
- All hormones in the serum
- Vitamins (e.g., vitamin B_{12}, vitamin D)
- Tumor markers in the serum, e.g., PSA, AFP, HCG, CEA, etc.

QUESTIONS

1. What is ELISA?
2. Write the principle of ELISA.
3. Mention various types of ELISA.
4. How is the ELISA test performed?
5. Write applications of ELISA.
6. What is the difference between indirect ELISA and sandwich ELISA?

EXPERIMENT 10

Immunodiffusion

COMPETENCY	LEARNING OBJECTIVES
BI11.16 Observe the use of commonly used equipments/ techniques in biochemistry laboratory including: pH meter, paper chromatography, protein electrophoresis, TLC, page, electrolyte analysis by ISE, ABG analyzer, ELISA, immunodiffusion, Autoanalyzer, quality control and DNA isolation from blood tissue.	1. Describe principle, types, and clinical application of immunodiffusion.

INTRODUCTION
Immunodiffusion is a technique/diagnostic test for the detection or measurement of antibodies and antigens by their precipitation. It involves diffusion through a substance, such as agar or agarose. Both agar and agarose are gelatin-like high-molecular-weight polysaccharides. Simply, it means precipitation in gel. It refers to any of the several techniques for obtaining a precipitate between an antibody and its specific antigen.

PRINCIPLE
Immunodiffusion techniques are based on specific antigen and antibody interactions. In which a solution containing specific antibody (test serum) is allowed to diffuse, through a semi-solid matrix (agar or agarose), towards another solution containing antigen. If the antibody recognizes the antigen, insoluble immune complexes form and will precipitate. This is visible as a line, ring or zone at the site of the antigen-antibody interactions. Presence of a precipitate is a positive test, which is used to detect and/or quantitate the antibody or antigen.

Precipitation reactions can be carried out in a test tube in a liquid state or in semisolid gels on a plate or in a tube. The reaction is more visible as a distinct band of precipitation in gel medium than in a liquid medium. It refers to any of the several techniques for obtaining a precipitate between an antibody and its specific antigen.

TYPES OF IMMUNODIFFUSION REACTION
Immunodiffusion reactions are classified based on the number of reactants diffusing and direction of diffusion as follows:
- Single diffusion in one dimension (Oudin procedure)
- Double diffusion in one dimension (Oakley Fulthorpe procedure)
- Single diffusion in two dimension (radial immunodiffusion or Mancini method)
- Double diffusion in two dimensions (Ouchterlony double immunodiffusion)

Single Diffusion in One Dimension (Oudin Procedure)

* As the name suggests, it is the single diffusion of antigen in a agar in one dimension.
* In this method, antibody is incorporated into agar gel in a test tube and the antigen solution is poured over it.
* The Ag diffuses downward through agar gel, and a line of precipitation is formed **(Figure 10.1)**.
* The number of precipitate band shows the number of different antigen present in antigen solution.

Double Diffusion in One Dimension (Oakley Fulthorpe Procedure)

* In this method, the antibody is incorporated in agar gel in a test tube above which a layer of plain agar is placed.
* The antigen is then layered on the top of this plain.
* During the course of time, the antigen and antibody move toward each other through the intervening layer of plain agar.
* In this zone of plain agar, both antigen and antibody react with each other to form a band of precipitation at their optimum concentration **(Figure 10.1)**.
* Single diffusion in two dimension (radial immunodiffusion or Mancini method)
* It is also called radial immunodiffusion. In this method, serum containing antibody is incorporated in agar gel on a slide or petri dish. The wells are cut on the surface of the gel.
* The antigen is then applied to the well cut into the gel. It diffuses radially from the well and reacts with antibody present in gel and forms ring-shaped bands of precipitation around the well **(Figure 10.2)**.
* The diameter of the ring is directly proportional to the concentration of the antigen.
* Radial immunodiffusion is used to measure IgG, IgM, IgA and complement components in the serum and antibodies to influenza virus in the sera.

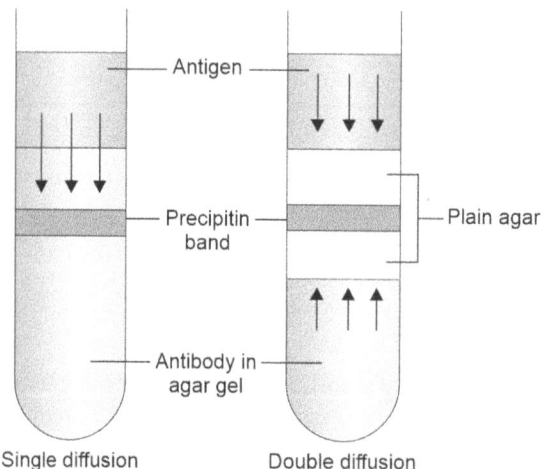

Figure 10.1: Single and double diffusion in one dimension.

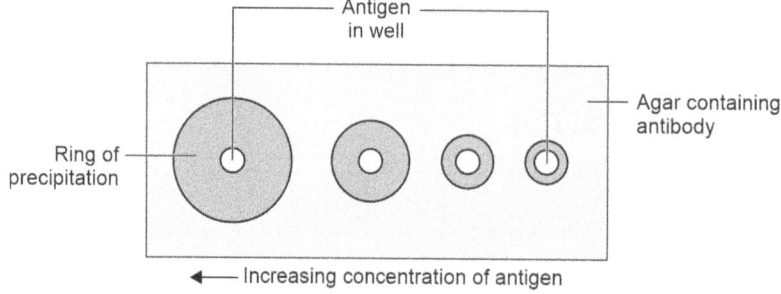

Figure 10.2: Radial immunodiffusion.

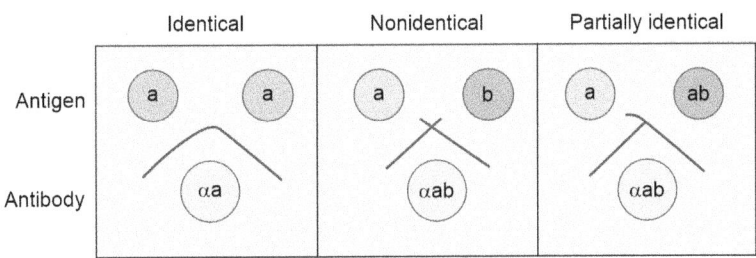

Figure 10.3: Double diffusion in two dimensions (Ouchterlony).

Double Diffusion in Two Dimensions (Ouchterlony Double Immunodiffusion)

❖ In this method, both the antigen and antibody diffuse independently through agar gel in two dimensions, horizontally and vertically.
❖ The test is performed by cutting wells in the agar gel poured on a glass slide or in a petri dish.
❖ The antiserum consisting of antibody is placed in the central well and different antigens are added to the wells surrounding the center well.
❖ If two adjacent antigens are identical, the lines of precipitate formed by antigen and antibody will fuse to form an **arc**. If they are unrelated, the lines will **cross each other**. If there is partial identity, there will be cross reaction with branch formation (**Figure 10.3**).

APPLICATIONS OF IMMUNODIFFUSION TECHNIQUE

❖ Immunodiffusion techniques are mostly used in immunology to determine the quantity or concentration of an antigen in a sample.
❖ Estimation of the immunoglobulin classes in sera.
❖ Estimation of IgG, IgM antibodies in sera to influenza viruses.
❖ To determine relative concentrations of antibodies in serum.
❖ To compare properties of two different antigens.
❖ To determine the relative purity of an antigen preparation

QUESTIONS

1. Write principle of immunodiffusion.
2. What are various types of immunodiffusion?
3. What is the difference between single diffusion and double immunodiffusion?
4. Write applications of immunodiffusion.

EXPERIMENT 11

DNA Isolation from Blood/Tissues

COMPETENCY	LEARNING OBJECTIVES
BI11.16 Observe the use of commonly used equipments/techniques in biochemistry laboratory including: pH meter, paper chromatography of amino acid, protein electrophoresis, TLC, PAGE, electrolyte analysis by ISE, ABG analyzer, ELISA, immunodiffusion, autoanalyzer, quality control and DNA isolation from blood/tissue.	1. Describe principle, methods and basic process of DNA isolation. 2. Describe use and application of the extracted DNA in different sectors.

INTRODUCTION

DNA isolation is a process of purification of DNA from sample using combination of physical and chemical methods. Isolation of DNA is needed for genetic analysis, which is used for scientific, medical, or forensic proposes. DNA can be isolated from any living or dead organism. Common sources for DNA isolation include whole blood, hair, sperm, bones, nails, tissues, blood stains, saliva, buccal swabs, epithelial cells, urine, cerebrospinal fluids, amniotic fluids, bacteria, animal tissues. Manual methods as well as commercially available kits are used for DNA extraction.

PRINCIPLE OF DNA ISOLATION

The basic principle of DNA isolation is disruption of the cell wall, cell membrane, and nuclear membrane to release the highly intact DNA into solution followed by precipitation of DNA and removal of the contaminating biomolecules, such as the proteins, polysaccharides, lipids, phenols, and other secondary metabolites by enzymatic or chemical methods.

METHODS OF DNA ISOLATION

For isolation of DNA from tissues, the tissue has to be homogenized by homogenizer in phosphate buffer saline (phosphate buffer with salt). DNA can be isolated by two methods:
1. Manual method: Phenol-chloroform extraction method
2. Commercial kit method

BASIC PROCESS OF DNA ISOLATION

For the isolation of DNA, there are various steps and methods involved. There basic steps for the extraction of DNA consists of four major steps:

1. **Lysis of the cells:** The nucleus and cell are broken first for the release of DNA. This is done by:
   - *Chemical method [Sodium Dodecyl Sulfate (SDS)]:* It has protein denaturing properties. So, it can be used in cleaning procedures and lysing cells during DNA extraction.
   - *Enzymatic method (Proteinase K):* It is a broad-spectrum serine protease enzyme. It digests protein and also inactivates nuclease enzyme which can degrade DNA or RNA during purification.
   - *Mechanical method (Mortar and pastel/grinding/blending/ultra-sonication/homogenization):* These mechanical methods apply force to separate out intracellular protein. This method is usually used for nucleic acid extraction from tissue in combination with chemical or enzyme in cell lysis step.
2. **Separation of DNA from the cellular debris:** After lysis, DNA has been freed from the nucleus but mixed with cell parts. A variety of procedures can be used to remove these contaminants, leaving the DNA in a pure form. The most commonly used procedures are:
   - **Phenol–Chloroform extraction:** Phenol denatures proteins in sample. After centrifugation of sample, denaturated proteins stay in organic phase while aqueous phase containing DNA is mixed with chloroform. The chloroform acts as a solvent and removes lipid.
   - **Minicolumn purification:** Minicolumn purification that relies on the fact that the nucleic acids may bind (adsorption) to the solid phase (silica or other) depending on the pH and the salt concentration of the buffer.
3. **Precipitation of DNA:** The supernatant, which contains DNA, is then mixed with ethanol or isopropanol, which causes the DNA to precipitate as it is insoluble in alcohol.
4. **Purification of DNA:** Now, the DNA has been separated from the aqueous phase due to precipitation. A small pellet of DNA can be collected by centrifugation. It is rinsed with alcohol for the removal of cellular debris and remaining unwanted materials. The purified DNA is redissolved in water (usually with a small amount of EDTA and buffer) for storage and use in other reactions.

Note that this process has purified DNA from a sample; if we want to further isolate a specific gene or DNA fragment, we must use additional techniques, such as **polymerase chain reaction** (**PCR**).

Phenol-Chloroform Extraction Method

A common way to isolate DNA is via the phenol-chloroform extraction method. This method is suitable for extracting DNA from various samples, including blood, suspension culture, and tissue. It produces relatively high yields and higher purity DNA than conventional extraction methods. Because this technique uses toxic chemicals, such as phenol, to denature proteins and chloroform to solubilize lipids, it should be performed in a fume hood, and the necessary precautions should be taken while handling.

- ❖ Like all DNA extraction methods, the phenol-chloroform process begins with destroying the cell membrane and non-nucleic acid cellular components **(Figure 11.1).**
- ❖ Cells are treated with a lysis buffer typically containing denaturing detergents, such as sodium dodecyl sulfate (SDS), and depending upon the type of DNA (e.g., genomic, mitochondrial, or plasmid), can include other additives. For instance, lysis buffers for extracting plasmid DNA from bacterial cells will contain sodium hydroxide for alkaline lysis and potassium acetate for the renaturation of the plasmid DNA.
- ❖ A mixture of phenolchloroformisoamyl alcohol (PCIA) is then added to the lysate to denature proteins and facilitate the precipitation of DNA. Since phenol is hydrophobic and less dense than water, centrifugation is used to partition the lysate into three distinct layers or phases.
- ❖ The bottom layer, or "organic phase," contains hydrophobic molecules, such as phenol, lipids, and chloroform. The middle layer, or "interphase," consists of denatured proteins, and the top layer, or "aqueous phase," comprises DNA and other polar molecules. The aqueous phase is then removed and transferred to a clean tube.
- ❖ When the aqueous phase is successfully transferred, DNA is precipitated using a solution of ammonium acetate and ethanol.
- ❖ The resulting DNA pellet is separated via centrifugation. Often, multiple ethanol washes are needed to remove contaminants and further concentrate the DNA.
- ❖ Each added wash involves removing the supernatant, re-suspending the pellet with ethanol, and centrifuging the tube. Following the final wash, the pellet is air-dried and re-suspended in a polar solution, such as an elution buffer.

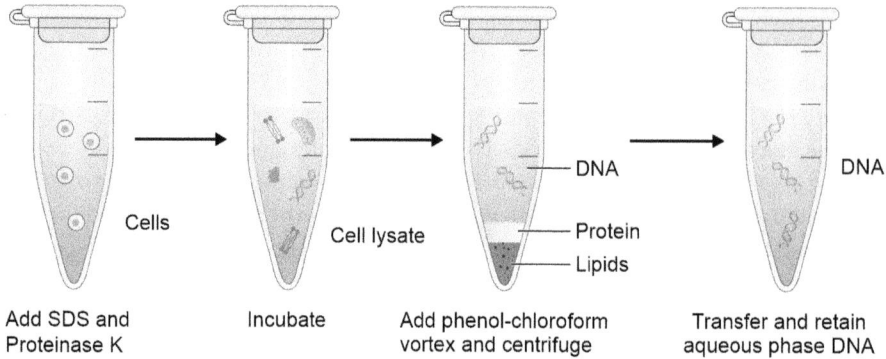

Figure 11.1: Extraction of DNA.

Uses and Applications of the Extracted DNA in Different Sectors

Below are some significant uses and applications of extracted DNA.
- **Forensics:** As DNA can be extracted from skin, hair or blood, DNA is used by forensic teams to determine if a person is a suspect. In addition, DNA proves someone's guilt or innocence. DNA extracted is used in the genetic fingerprinting process.
- **DNA paternity test:** DNA extraction is helpful in the determination of the paternity of a child.
- **Ancestry tracking:** DNA analysis is necessary to know about the ancestors of a person.
- **Medical tests:** DNA extraction is necessary for diagnosing genetic diseases. DNA is also useful to identify whether a person is a carrier of the disease, even if there is no symptom of the disease. Isolation of nucleic acid (DNA or RNA) is a key preliminary step in any molecular diagnostic procedure.
- **Genetic engineering:** The extracted DNA is useful for the genetic engineering in cloning of gene.

QUESTIONS

1. What is the basic principle of DNA isolation?
2. Write basic steps of DNA extraction.
3. What are the materials required for DNA isolation?
4. Write uses and applications of DNA isolation.

EXPERIMENT 12

Autoanalyzer

COMPETENCY	LEARNING OBJECTIVES
BI11.16 Observe the use of commonly used equipments/ techniques in biochemistry laboratory including: pH meter, paper chromatography of amino acid, protein electrophoresis, TLC, PAGE, electrolyte analysis by ISE, ABG analyzer, ELISA, immunodiffusion, autoanalyser, quality control and DNA isolation from blood/tissue.	1. Describe the basic components, principle, and advantages of semi-automated biochemistry analyzer. 2. Describe the basic components, principle, and advantages of fully-automated biochemistry analyzer.

INTRODUCTION

A biochemistry analyzer is a clinical chemical analyzer machine that measures the biochemical components of biological sample, such as blood, urine, plasma, and so on. While initially, this process was carried out manually by lab technicians and analysts, it gradually became tedious enough to cause hindrances. To avoid the delay in delivering test results for each sample, the need for an analyzing machine was registered.

AUTOANALYZER

Autoanalyzer is an automated analyzer in a clinical laboratory designed to analyze various biochemical tests quickly, with minimal human assistance. Automation of the testing process has reduced; slow, clumsy, and error-prone manual methods of analysis. Samples used in the analyzers include; blood, serum, plasma, urine, cerebrospinal fluid, and other fluids from within the body.

Principle of Autoanalyzer

Automated biochemistry analyzers based on photoelectric colorimetric principle to measure a specific chemical composition in body fluids. According to the degree of automation of the instrument, it is divided into:
- Semi-automated biochemical analyzers
- Fully automated biochemical analyzers.

Semi-autoanalyzer VS fully automatic biochemistry analyzer is given in **Table 12.1**.

SEMI-AUTOMATED BIOCHEMISTRY ANALYZERS

Semi-autoanalyzers are suitable for laboratories which have moderate amount of work load. These analyzers are called semi-autoanalyzers (*see* **Figure 1.17**), because the initial stages of a sample analysis are performed externally/manually by laboratory technicians, such as:
- Pipetting of reagent
- Pipetting of samples
- Mixing and incubating the reaction mixture

Rests of the procedure given below are performed by the semi-autoanalyzers:
- Setting of incubation temperature (for kinetic determinations)
- Zero setting
- Reading light intensities (absorbance) of end product
- Calculating test results
- Displaying test results
- Printing test results
- Storage/memorizing of results

Components of Semi-Auto Biochemistry Analyzer

- **Color filter:** Different colored filters are present in the machine which signifies different wavelengths. The common wavelengths of filters include 340 nm, 405 nm, 500 nm, 546 nm, 578 nm, 620 nm, and 670 nm.
- **Light source:** The most common light source is the halogen light. In some models, the light source can also be a LED light.
- **Photo-detector:** Photo-detector measures the absorbance (optical density) of the sample solution.
- **Flow cell/Cuvette:** It is for the storage of the sample.
- **Temperature controller** Have the settings of temperature at 25°C, 6°C, and 37°C.
- **Pumping system:** A pump draws the sample from the sipping tube to the flow cell. Once the measurement is completed, it again draws the fluid out of the flow cell.
- **Incubator:** Inbuilt incubator for holding a few test tubes.
- **Thermal printer:** There is an inbuilt thermal printer at the top of the machine.
- **Fan:** They are necessary to maintain the set temperature and to cool the machine.
- **Display:** It is generally LCD type with/without a touch screen.

Use of Semi auto Biochemistry Analyzer

Semi auto biochemistry analyzer is capable to perform tests on whole blood, serum, plasma, cerebrospinal fluid and urine. It is capable of performing routine biochemistry, hormonal assay, electrolytes, and enzyme investigations.

Table 12.1: Semi-autoanalyzer VS fully automatic biochemistry analyzer.

Function	Fully automatic analyzer	Semi-autoanalyzer
Sampling	Automatic addition of sample	Manual addition of samples
Number of samples analyzed	200-300 samples each time	Limited capacity to handle workload
Measurement time	Generally 2 hours, the number of 200 samples, each sample size detection time of 0.6 seconds	Time consuming. 5–6 minutes per sample size
Cleaning function	Automatic cleaning	Manual cleaning
Difference of sample volume	Multiple samples at a time	One sample at a time
Human error	Manual intervention less or even no manual intervention, reducing human error	Lot of human intervention and hence more errors
Quality control data analysis	Available	Not available

FULLY-AUTOMATED BIOCHEMISTRY ANALYZERS

The fully-automatic biochemical analyzer (*see* **Figure 1.18**) is fully automated from sample addition to result generation. All functions, such as the steps of sampling, adding reagents, mixing, incubation, automatic detection, calculation of results, data processing and printing, and cleaning after the experiment are performed by machine. The operator only needs to put the sample on the specific position of the analyzer and choose the program to start the instrument to take the test report.

Fully automated analyzers are of two types:
1. Batch analyzers
2. Random access analyzers:
   - Batch analyzers performed only one type of test at a time. Various batches of the samples are made. For example, batch of glucose, batch of urea, etc. the biggest disadvantage of these analyzers was that they were not patient oriented and so became outdated.
   - Random access analyzers: These analyzers complete all tests on one sample hence are patient oriented. These analyzers are currently in use.

Component of Autoanalyzer (Figure 12.1)

- **Sampler**: Aspirates samples, standards, wash solutions into the system.
- **Proportioning pump**: Mixes samples with the reagents so that proper chemical color reactions can take place, which are then read by the colorimeter.
- **Dialyzer**: Separates interfacing substances from the sample by permitting selective passage of sample components through a semipermeable membrane.
- **Heating bath**: Controls temperature (typically at 37 °C), as temperature is critical in color development
- **Colorimeter**: Monitors the changes in optical density of the fluid stream flowing through a tubular flow cell. Color intensities proportional to the substance concentrations are converted to equivalent electrical voltages.
- **Recorder:** Displays the output information in a graphical form.

Functioning of Autoanalyzers

- The flow of the analytical stream is directed through plastic tubing from one module to another by air bubbles.
- The samples are loaded into the cup of the sampler and the channels of the proportionating pump aspirate them as well as dilute them.
- The diluted serum samples are led through one of the dialyzer unit.
- The pump introduces suitable reagents through the other side of the dialyzer.
- The two streams run side-by-side being separated only by dialyzing membrane.
- A portion of dialyzable constituents of serum passes across the membrane to the reagent stream.
- Further treatment like incubation at suitable temperature is given in the constant temperature heating bath.

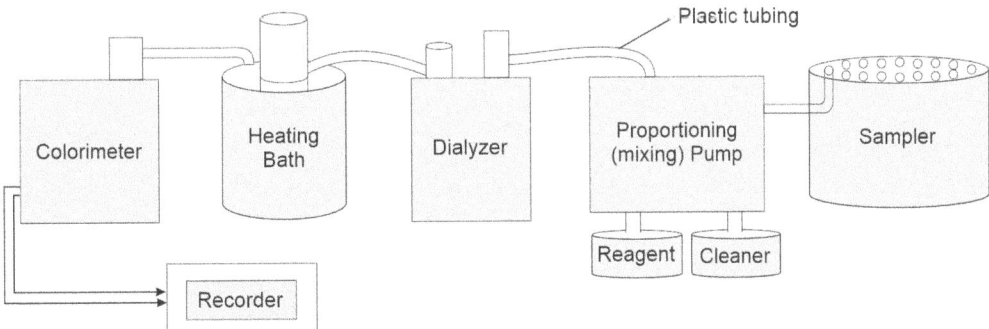

Figure 12.1: Components of autoanalyzer.

- The intensity of the color developed is measured in a colorimeter and recorded in the recorder.
- Suitable standards are treated in the same way.

Advantages of Autoanalyzers
- Large number of samples can be tested in short time.
- Large workload can be handled without comparable increase in laboratory staff.
- Contact with the sample and reagent is less as compared to the manual method.
- Tests performed on autoanalyzers are much more accurate, precise, sensitive and specific as compared to manual methods.
- Internal and external quality programs can be implemented efficiently and effectively by using autoanalyzers.

QUESTIONS
1. What is autoanalyzer? Write the different types of autoanalyzer.
2. What is semi-automated analyzer?
3. What is a fully automated analyzer?
4. Write difference between semi- and fully-automated analyzer?
5. Write the advantages of autoanalyzers?

EXPERIMENT 13

Protein Electrophoresis and PAGE

COMPETENCY	LEARNING OBJECTIVES
BI11.16 Observe the use of commonly used equipments/techniques in biochemistry laboratory including: pH meter, paper chromatography of amino acid, protein electrophoresis, TLC, PAGE, electrolyte analysis by ISE, ABG analyzer, ELISA, immunodiffusion, autoanalyzer, quality control and DNA isolation from blood/tissue.	1. Describe electrophoresis: Definition, principle, types and applications. 2. Describe components of electrophoresis apparatus. 3. Describe types of support medium and factors affecting electrophoretic mobility. 4. Describe separation of serum proteins by agarose gel electrophoresis and its clinical importance. 5. Describe polyacrylamide gel electrophoresis (PAGE): Principle and its applications.

INTRODUCTION

Electrophoresis is a general term that describes the migration and separation of charged particles (ions) in a **supporting medium** under the influence of an **electric field**. Different types of supporting media, such as Whatman filter paper, membrane of cellulose acetate, agarose gel, and polyacrylamide gel are used.

ELECTROPHORESIS

Definition

Electrophoresis is a laboratory technique used to separate DNA, RNA or protein molecules based on their size, shape and electrical charge. An electric current is used to move the molecules through a supporting medium.

Principle

Any charged ion or molecule when placed in an electric field move towards the negative or positive electrodes based on their charge. Negatively charged ions or molecules are migrated to the positive electrode (anode), while positively charged species are migrated to the negative electrode (cathode). For example, proteins and nucleic acids have negative charge and therefore they migrate towards the anode.

Types of Electrophoresis

Depending upon the mode of operation and separation, electrophoresis is classified into various types:

1. Moving Boundary Electrophoresis

Moving boundary electrophoresis involves the migration of charged molecules in a free moving solution, without the presence of a supporting medium. This method is rarely used.

2. Zone Electrophoresis

This is the most common type of electrophoresis. In zone electrophoresis, the sample is applied as a spot or band on chemically inert and homogenous supporting medium on which the separation of the components takes place in the form of zones or bands. Depending on support medium used for separation, zone electrophoresis is further classified as:
- **Paper electrophoresis:** Supporting medium is Whatman filter paper
- **Cellulose acetate electrophoresis:** Supporting medium is membrane of cellulose acetate
- **Agarose gel electrophoresis:** Supporting medium is agarose gel
- **Polyacrylamide gel electrophoresis (PAGE):** Supporting medium is polyacrylamide gel

Applications of Electrophoresis

- The electrophoresis procedure is used in clinical laboratory for separation of **serum proteins** (for diagnosis of various protein-related disorders), lipoproteins, isoenzymes, hemoglobin (in diseases like sickle cell anemia and thalassemia) and RNA and DNA.
- Immunoelectrophoresis is used to determine specific classes of immunoglobulins.
- Western blotting is a laboratory technique used to detect a specific protein/antibody in a blood or tissue sample. The method first make use of gel electrophoresis to separate the sample's proteins.
- Southern blot techniques to identify specific nucleic acid sequences (DNA or RNA) used for prenatal diagnosis of inborn errors, diagnosis of viral infections and identification of risk factors for cancer is also based on electrophoretic principle.

COMPONENTS OF ELECTROPHORESIS APPARATUS

Electrophoresis is carried out in a tank suitable for supporting medium. Supporting medium may be Whatman filter paper, membrane of cellulose acetate, agarose gel, and polyacrylamide gel, etc. General components of electrophoresis apparatus include (**Figure 13.1**)
- **Buffer tank:** Carries buffer. Buffer functions to carry the current and maintain the pH of the medium.
- **Support medium:** Provide the matrix in which separation takes place.
- **Wicks:** Connects support medium with buffer to complete the circuit.
- **Power pack:** Provides an electrical field for the movement of charged particles.
- **Electrodes:** Anode and cathode
- **Cover:** Reduces evaporation of buffer and prevents contamination during the electrophoretic run.
- **Densitometer:** For quantification of separated bands.

TYPES OF SUPPORT MEDIUM AND FACTORS AFFECTING ELECTROPHORETIC MOBILITY

Different types of support medium and buffers are utilized to separate different types of molecules.
- **Whatman filter paper:** Whatman's filter paper is used as a support medium. As it requires long run-time (12–16 hours) and low voltage for separation, the resolution is poor due to the increased diffusion of separated analytes.
- **Cellulose acetate:** Cellulose acetate membrane is one of the preferred solid media as it requires less run-time (<1 hour). Due to this, the resolution of separated bands is far superior to paper electrophoresis. It is widely used for separating lipoproteins, proteins, isoenzyme, and hemoglobin variants.

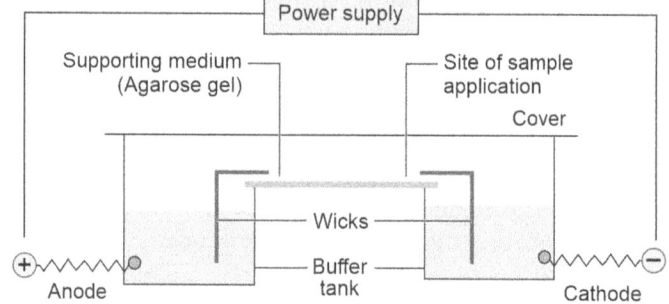

Figure 13.1: Components of electrophoresis apparatus.

❖ **Agarose gel:** Agarose is a type of heteropolysaccharide. It forms a viscous solution when dissolved in a hot buffer solution (50-55 °C), but it solidifies as a gel on cooling down. It is used to separate serum proteins, hemoglobin, nucleic acids, polymerase chain reaction products, etc.
❖ **Polyacrylamide gel:** Acrylamide is used to make polyacrylamide gel. Acrylamide is soluble in water and upon addition of water it polymerizes resulting in formation of **polyacrylamide gel.** This gel can be used for a wide variety of analytes, such as proteins, peptides, nucleic acid, nucleotides, etc.

Factors Affecting Electrophoretic Mobility

The rate and direction of particle movement in an electric field depends on the:
1. Net charge of the molecules
2. Size and shape of the molecules
3. Strength of the electrical field
4. Support medium properties
5. Ionic strength of the buffer
6. Temperature

❖ **Size, shape, and net charge of the molecule:** Mobility is inversely proportional to the size of the molecule and directly proportional to the net charge of the molecule.
❖ **Strength of the electrical field:** Mobility is directly proportional to voltage.
❖ **Buffer:** Buffer functions to carry the current and maintain the pH of the medium. The optimum ionic strength of the buffer is necessary as higher ionic strength increases the share of current carried by buffer ions and slows down the sample migration. It also produces a high amount of heat, leading to increased diffusion of separation of bands. While low ionic strength of the buffer also reduces resolution due to reduced overall current passing through the medium. The ionization of molecules, such as proteins, amino acids, etc., depends on the pH of the medium. Alteraiton in the pH of the medium can alter the direction and velocity of migration.
❖ **Supporting medium:** If medium having affinity for the molecules in samples, can delay the rate of migration and can decrease the resolution of separation. The pore size in the support medium is inversely proportional to the concentration of gel. Adjusting pore size according to the properties of a molecule of interest is necessary for optimum resolution.

SEPARATION OF SERUM PROTEINS BY AGAROSE GEL ELECTROPHORESIS

Principle

Proteins at alkaline pH (8.6) bears negative charge and migrate towards the anode in an electric field. Different serum proteins (**albumin** and **globulins**) are separated during the migration due to their different mobility based on charge to size ratio.

❖ **By agarose gel electrophoresis** serum proteins are separated into five fractions based on their electrophoretic mobility. Albumins represent the largest fraction and the remaining fractions are five types of globulins; α_1-**globulin,** α_2-**globulin,** β_1-**globulin,** β_2-**globulin** and γ-**globulin.**
  - Albumin having high negative charge and low molecular weight, migrate towards the positive anode.
  - Whereas γ-globulins that having the greatest molecular weight and the lowest negative charge is closer to the cathode.
❖ When the electrophoresis process is completed, a **densitogram (proteinogram)** is plotted with a densitometer. Densitogram shows several peaks representing individual protein fractions and their concentrations in serum. The first peak is the largest and represents **albumins**, and the next four peaks represent globulins α_1, α_2, β, and γ **(Figure 13.2).**

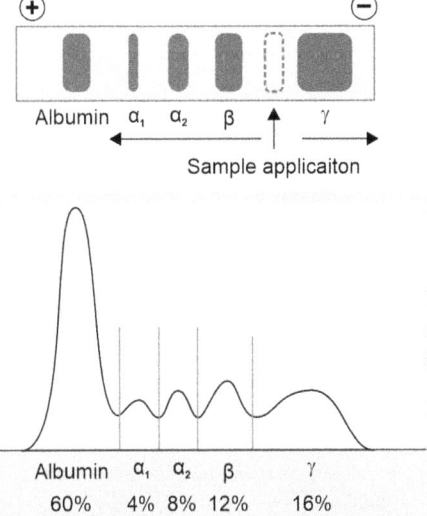

Figure 13.2: Normal serum protein electrophoretic pattern.

- **Albumins** are the largest protein component in serum. Albumin is usually a single protein.
- α_1 **globulins** represent the smallest group of serum proteins. This fraction contains the α_1 **antitrypsin** (protease inhibitor, acute-phase protein), which represents more than 90% of the α_1 fraction, α_1-**chymotrypsin**, α_1 **fetoprotein**, **thyroxine binding globulin (TBG)** and **high density lipoprotein, HDL**.
- α_2 **Globulins**: The most important α_2 globulins include the copper transporter **ceruloplasmin**, α_2 **macroglobulin** and **haptoglobin**.
- **β- globulins:** The β fraction is divided into β_1 and β_2, but only one peak can be seen on the proteinogram.
    - β_1 globulins include the iron transporter **transferrin** and **low-density lipoprotein (LDL)**,
    - β_2 globulins include β_2 **microglobulin** and **complement proteins C3** and **C4**
- The γ globulin contains immunoglobulins (IgG, IgA, IgM, IgD and IgE).
- When plasma is used in the place of serum for protein electrophoresis, **fibrinogen** present in plasma appears in the β_2 region: Between the β and γ peaks, there is a so-called intermediate zone. C-reactive protein (CRP) accumulates in this part, and immunoglobulins (IgA and IgM) can also be found. In patients with liver cirrhosis, **β-γ bridge** can form that connects both peaks (**Figure 13.3**).

Clinical Importance of Serum Protein Electrophoresis

Serum protein electrophoretic patterns provide useful diagnostic information. In clinical practice, serum protein electrophoresis is suggested when multiple myeloma, macroglobulinemia, amyloidosis, or other protein disorders, such as acute and chronic inflammations, nephropathy, liver diseases, etc., is suspected.

❖ **Low levels of albumin** (hypoalbuminemia) are clinically significant. **Hypoalbuminemia** indicates either a **poor dietary intake (malnutrition)** or a **decreased synthesis** or an **increased loss**.
- **Chronic liver disease (liver cirrhosis)** is a common clinical condition associated with decreased albumin production. Synthesis of albumin occurs exclusively in liver (**Figure 13.3**).
- **Chronic kidney disease (CKD)** is the most common cause associated with an increased loss **of albumin** in urine (proteinuria). This clinical condition is known as **nephropathy (Figure 13.4)**.

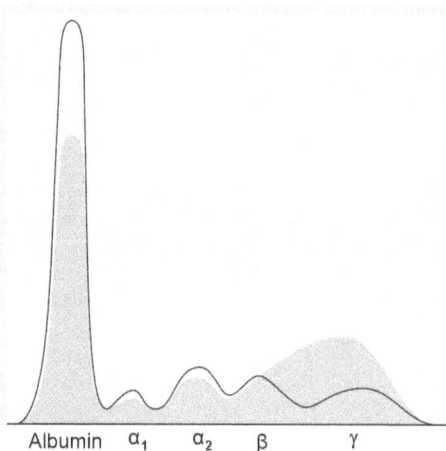

Figure 13.3: Electrophoretic pattern in liver cirrhosis.
- **Decrese in albumin:** Impaired liver function reduces the ability to synthesize proteins.
- **Reduced α_1 and α_2 fractions**
- **β-γ Bridge formation:** Due to the increased concentration of IgA
- **Polyclonal hypergammaglobulinemia:** In addition to IgA, other immunoglobulins are also elevated.

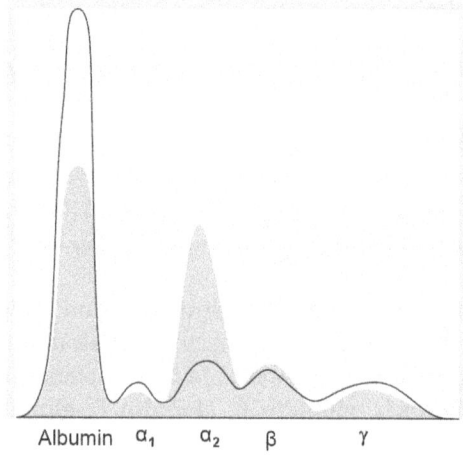

Figure 13.4: Electrophoretic pattern in nephrotic syndrome.
- **Decrese in albumin:** The damage to the glomeruli results in a greater loss of urine protein. If damage is to a lesser extent, only albumins (smaller molecules) are lost.
- **Reduced α_1 fractions**
- **Increase in α_2-globulins:** Due to increase in α_2-macroglobulin
- **Slight increase in β-globulin:** Due to increase in LDL level (may be related to the urinary loss of plasma albumin).
- **Decrease in the γ-globulin:** If damage is more, IgG is also lost.

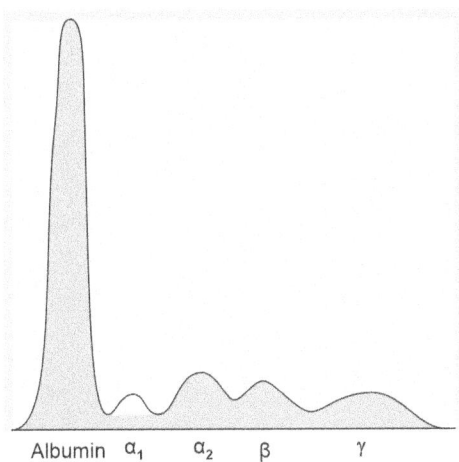

Figure 13.5: Electrophoretic pattern in α₁ antitrypsin deficiency.
* **Decreased α₁-globulin:** Decreased fraction of α₁ antitrypsin.

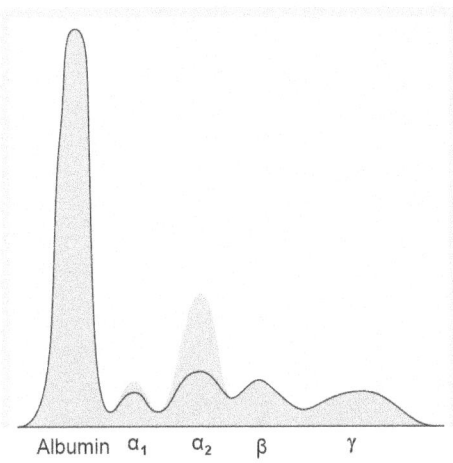

Figure 13.6: Electrophoretic pattern in acute inflammation.
* **Albumin** is normal or decreased.
* **Increase in α₁ and α₂-globulin:** Due to increase in acute-phase proteins.

❖ **Decreased α_1- globulin** is associated with α_1- **antitrypsin deficiency (Figure 13.5),** decreased globulin synthesis due to **liver disease**, or due to **urinary protein loss** in damaged kidney.

❖ An **increased** α_1-**globulin** band is observed in conditions of **inflammation (Figure 13.6)** due to increase in concentration of α_1-**antitrypsin** (acute-phase reactant)

❖ An **increased** α_2-**globulin band** observed in:
- **Acute inflammatory states** due to increased level of haptoglobin (acute-phase reactants) **(Figure 13.6).** The acute inflammatory response occurs as a result of infection, necrosis, burns, heart attack, injury, or after surgery.
- **Nephrotic syndrome (Figure 13.4)** due to increased α_2-**macroglobulin.** The elevation of α_2 macroglobulin is distinctly evident in nephritic syndrome, since it is a bulky molecule, and hence retained in circulation to compensate for the loss of other proteins in urine.

❖ Increased γ-globulin **(hypergammaglobulinemia)** is due to abnormal proliferation of the **lymphoid cells** producing immunoglobulins. Increased γ-globulin occurs in many malignant diseases, or liver cirrhosis **(Figure 13.3).** Hypergammaglobulinemia may be **monoclonal, polyclonal,** or **oligoclonal.**

❖ Monoclonal peak (M-peak) has only **one peak (Figure 13.7).** It is characteristic of malignant diseases that originate from only one malignant plasma cell clone. These secrete either one type of intact immunoglobulin, a heavy or light chain (Bence Jones protein), or a combination of these components. These proteins are called **para-proteins** or **M (monoclonal)** proteins. Common clinical disorders producing "M" Band in serum protein electrophoresis include **multiple myeloma** and **plasmacytoma** (tumor of plasma cells) and **Waldenstrom's Macroglobulinemia, lymphomas,** and **leukemia.**

❖ Polyclonal peak is broad/extended type **(Figure 13.8).** It originates from many plasma cell clones, which leads to an increase in serum concentration of several types of

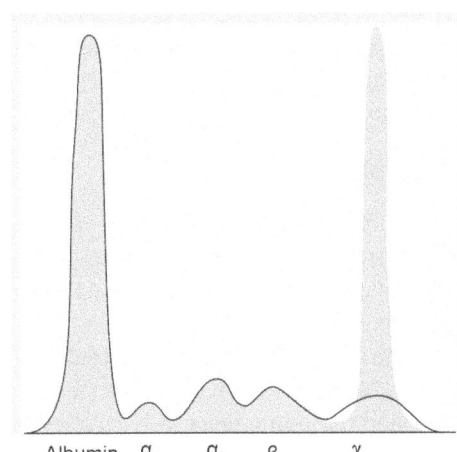

Figure 13.7: Monoclonal M peak in γ region.
* Increased γ-globulin has only one peak of monoclonal protein due to abnormal proliferation of the lymphoid cells producing one type of immunoglobulin.

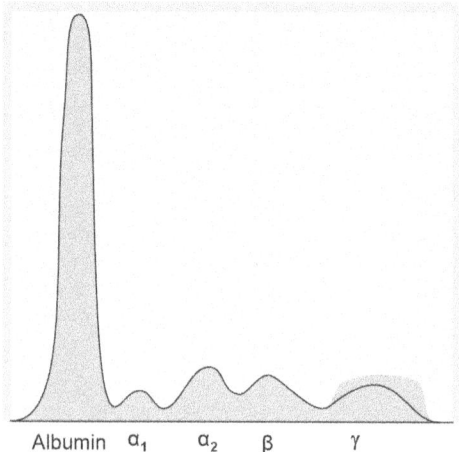

Figure 13.8: Polyclonal broad/extended type peak in γ fraction.
* Increased γ-globulin has broad/extended type peak due to increase concentration of several types of immunoglobulin.

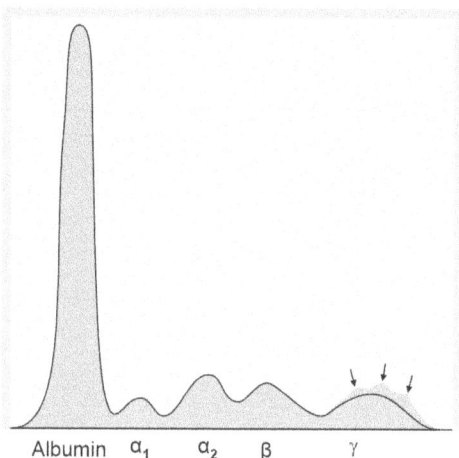

Figure 13.9: Oligoclonal band in γ fraction.
* Increased γ-globulin has more than two peaks.

immunoglobulin. Polyclonal peak commonly occurs in **chronic inflammation, infections, chronic liver diseases (cirrhosis), chronic kidney diseases**, etc.
* The oligoclonal peak has **more than two peaks** in the gamma region (**Figure 13.9**). This pattern occurs rarely with autoimmune disorders, amyloidosis, etc.

POLYACRYLAMIDE GEL ELECTROPHORESIS

In polyacrylamide gel electrophoresis (PAGE) **polyacrylamide gel** is used as the support media. It is widely used in **biochemistry, forensic chemistry, genetics, molecular biology** and **biotechnology** to separate biological macromolecules, usually **proteins** or **nucleic acids.**

Acrylamide is used to make polyacrylamide gel. Acrylamide is soluble in water and upon addition of water it polymerizes resulting in formation of **polyacrylamide gel.**

The basic principle of PAGE is to separate analytes by passing them through the pores of a polyacrylamide gel using an electric current. The small molecules can enter the pores and travel through the gel while large molecules get trapped at the pore openings.

Principle of PAGE

* Polyacrylamide gel electrophoresis (PAGE) is a technique used to separate proteins on the basis of their **size**. Electrophoretic separation of proteins on the basis of their size/molecular weight is possible only if the charge of all the protein molecules can be manipulated to the same sign. In such a case, the mobility of the protein molecules will be exclusively dependent on their size.
* In PAGE, an anionic **sodium dodecyl sulfate (SDS)** is used to bind to proteins to give them a negative charge. If protein solution is boiled briefly in the presence of sodium dodecyl sulfate (SDS), proteins in the solution get denatured, and transformed them into negatively charged linear polypeptide chains which masks the native charge of the protein. In this condition, electrophoretic mobility will depend on the number of amino acids and size/molecular weight of the polypeptide chains.
* Proteins are then separated according to their size/molecular weight using polyacrylamide gel in an electric field. When electric current is applied, proteins migrate through the gel to the positive electrode as they have a negative charge.
* Each molecule moves at a different rate based on its size/molecular weight—small molecules move more rapidly through the gel than larger ones and thus the all protein molecules are separated by size (**Figure 13.10**).

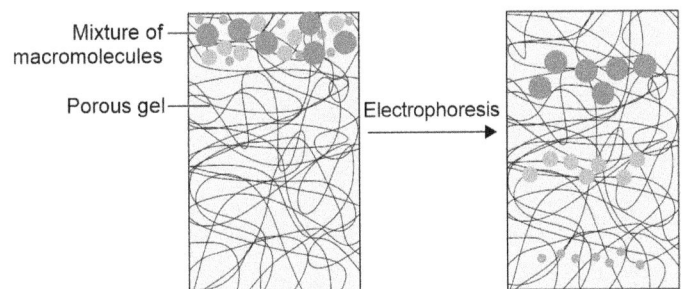

Figure 13.10: Separation of protein molecules according to their size by PAGE.

- Once electrophoresis is complete, the gel can be stained by a colored dye; **Coomassie Brilliant Blue** or **ethidium bromide** to make the separated proteins appear as distinct colored bands on the gel.
- After the visualization by a staining technique, the size of a protein can be calculated by comparing its migration distance with that of a known molecular weight proteins.
- The proteins can also be quantified as the protein content is directly proportional to the quantity of the bound dye.

Applications of PAGE

Polyacrylamide gel electrophoresis (PAGE) is a technique widely used in **biochemistry, forensic chemistry, genetics, molecular biology** and **biotechnology** to separate biological macromolecules, usually **proteins** or **nucleic acids.**
- It is used to measure the molecular weight and the size of the protein molecules.
- It is used to estimate the purity of the proteins.
- It is used in Western Blot technique which is used to detect a specific protein in a blood or tissue sample. In Western Blot sample's proteins are first separated by PAGE. The separated proteins are then detected by Western Blotting. For example, in the HIV test, HIV proteins are separated by SDS-PAGE and subsequently detected by Western Blot.
- Likewise it is used in Southern blots (used to detect specific DNA sequences) and Northern blots a (used to detect specific RNA sequences) for the separation of DNA and RNA.
- PAGE is used for **peptide mapping**. Peptide mapping is a technique to identify or verify a protein's primary structure (amino acid sequence and chemical modifications).

QUESTIONS

1. Define electrophoresis. Give its principle.
2. Give different types of electrophoresis.
3. Write factor affecting electrophoretic mobility and types of support medium.
4. Write different components of electrophoresis apparatus
5. Draw normal electrophoretic pattern of serum protein separated by agarose gel electrophoresis with its proteinogram.
6. Draw different proteinogram associated with various disorders compared with normal.
7. Write the principle of PAGE.
8. Write applications of PAGE.

EXPERIMENT 14

Paper Chromatography of Amino Acids and TLC

COMPETENCY	LEARNING OBJECTIVES
BI11.16 Observe the use of commonly used equipments/techniques in biochemistry laboratory including: pH meter, paper chromatography of amino acid, protein electrophoresis, TLC, PAGE, electrolyte analysis by ISE, ABG analyzer, ELISA, immunodiffusion, autoanalyzer, quality control and DNA isolation from blood/tissue.	1. Describe principle and types of chromatography. 2. Describe separation of amino acids by paper chromatography and its applications. 3. Describe thin layer chromatography and its applications.

INTRODUCTION

Chromatography is an analytical technique that enables the separation, identification, and purification of the components of a mixture for qualitative and quantitative analysis.

PRINCIPLE AND TYPES OF CHROMATOGRAPHY

Principle

A mixture is separated by distributing its components between two phases (stationary phase and mobile phase). The stationary phase remains fixed in place while the mobile phase carries the components of the mixture through the medium being used. The separation of components depends on the relative affinity of components towards both the phases. The components which have a higher affinity to the stationary phase move slowly while the other components travel fast and facilitate the separation of the components within that mixture. On completion of the separation process, their character and nature are identified by suitable detection techniques.

Types of Chromatography

Chromatographic methods are generally classified according to the physical state of the mobile phase—**liquid chromatography** and **gas chromatography (Figure 14.1).** This is further sub-classified according to how the stationary phase is contained for a particular chromatographic method. For example, liquid chromatography is divided into **flat/planar** and **column** methods. In flat chromatography, the thin layer of stationary phase is mechanically supported on a sheet of paper or glass or plastic and in column chromatography it is packed into glass or metal columns.

EXPERIMENT 14: Paper Chromatography of Amino Acids and TLC

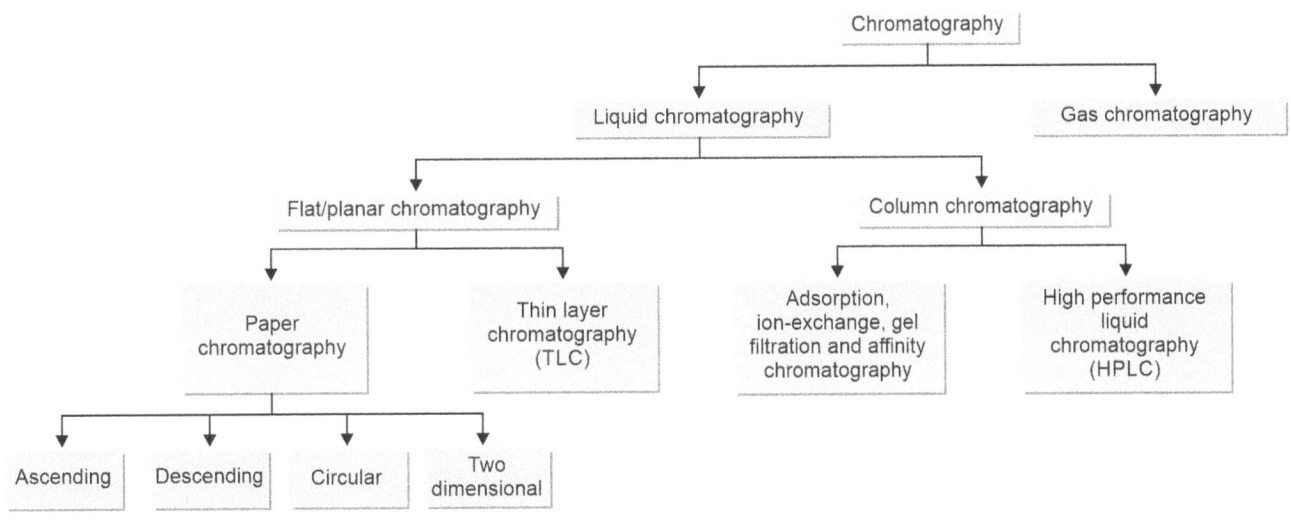

Figure 14.1: Types of chromatography.

SEPARATION OF AMINO ACIDS BY PAPER CHROMATOGRAPHY AND ITS APPLICATION

Paper chromatography is a type of liquid/planar/partition chromatography whereby chromatography procedures are run on a specialized paper. The paper acts as solid supporting medium.

There are different modes in which paper chromatography is carried out; these are:
- **Ascending paper chromatography:** The solvent moves in an upward direction.
- **Descending paper chromatography:** The movement of the flow of solvent is downwards.
- **Radial or circular paper chromatography:** Circular shape paper is taken and materials to be analyzed are placed at the center of the circular filter paper.
- **Two dimensional paper chromatography:** Substances which have the same Rf values can be resolved with the help of two-dimensional paper chromatography.

Principle Paper Chromatography

In paper chromatography, Whatman no 1 filter paper sheets acts as a support medium. Components which are to be separated are distributed between a stationary phase and a mobile phase. Here, stationary phase is water that is adsorbed within the pores of Whatman no 1 filter paper and the organic solvent is the mobile phase that travels along with the filter paper. The paper serves as a support to hold the stationary phase of the solvent system. Components of the sample are separated due to the differences in their affinities towards the stationary phase (water) and mobile phase when traveling through capillary action between the pores of the filter paper. Compounds which are more soluble in the organic phase move faster.

Requirements

- **Supporting medium:** Whatman no 1 filter paper
- Standard amino acids
- **Amino acid mixture to be separated:** For example, glycine and leucine
- **Solvent:** n-Butanol: acetic acid: distilled water in the ratio of 4:1:5 respectively
- 1% Ninhydrin solution

Procedure

- Take a sheet of Whatman's filter paper no. 1 and cut it into an appropriate size. Make a baseline 2.5 cm above one end of paper. Now make points on line at equal distance. In the diagram, the points are labeled 1, 2, 3, 4, and 5 for known amino acids and M for unknown mixture of amino acids.
- Take 100 mL of solvent (n-Butanol: acetic acid: distilled water) in chromatography tank.

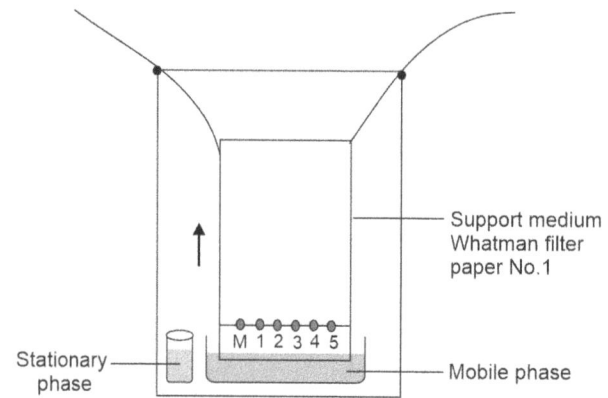

Figure 14.2: Paper chromatography: Ascending paper chromatography.

- Apply 1-2 μL of various amino acid and mixture solutions at each point.
- Gently fix other end of the filter paper with clip or thread at top end of tank. The lower end of paper on which the samples have been applied should dip into the solvent and solvent is allowed to flow past the spot of the application **(Figure 14.2)**.
- Water that is held within the pores of filter paper is the stationary phase and the organic solvent which moves over the paper is the mobile phase. Compounds which are more soluble in the organic phase move faster. Leave the tank undisturbed for one hour so that the solvent migrates up to the upper end of strip.
- Remove the paper and mark the solvent front with pencil and dry it in oven at 100-110°C for 10 to 15 minutes. The spots are still invisible (**Figure 14.3**). Spray the Ninhydrin solution on the strip and dry them again. Ninhydrin reacts with amino acids to give colored compounds, mainly brown or purple. Appearance of purple spots indicates the position of amino acids (**Figure 14.3**).
- The spots are marked and Rf (retention factor) value is determined. The ratio of the distance moved by compound to that moved by the solvent is known as Rf (**Figure 14.4**). Rf value is used to identify particular amino acids in the mixture during the chromatographic separation. Thus, after separation, the Rf value is calculated for each amino acid and identified by comparing it with the standard Rf value chart.
- In the given experiment, you can easily compare the spots in the mixture with those of the known amino acids, both from their positions and their colors as shown in **Figure 14.3**.

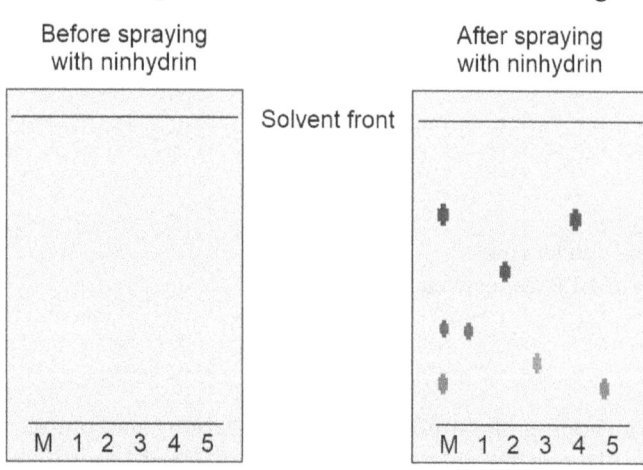

Figure 14.3: Separation of amino acids by paper chromatography.

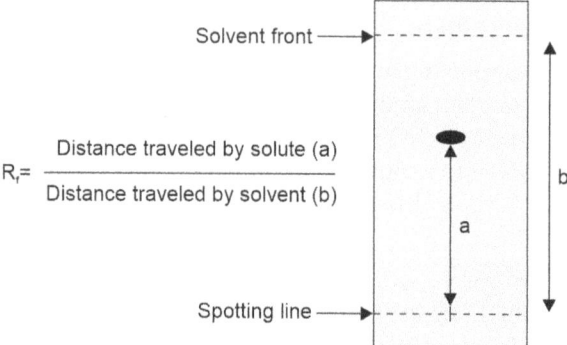

Figure 14.4: Retention factor calculations.

Application of Paper Chromatography

- Paper chromatography is used in the biological separation of amino acids, peptides, alkaloids, sugars, lipids, etc.
- Clinically paper chromatography is used for screening of urine for some inborn errors of metabolism. For example, paper chromatography is used for identification of type of amino aciduria like cystinuria, phenylketonuria, glycinuria, etc.
- It is an essential tool in forensic science. It is routinely used to identify and compare samples of drugs, explosives, inks (to check at a bank for forgery) and biological samples, such as saliva, urine, blood and other.
- Paper chromatography is used to detect the contaminants in foods and drinks.
- Assessment of the level of pollutants in the water supply can be determined using paper chromatography.
- Paper chromatography is also used to detect alcohol levels in the blood.

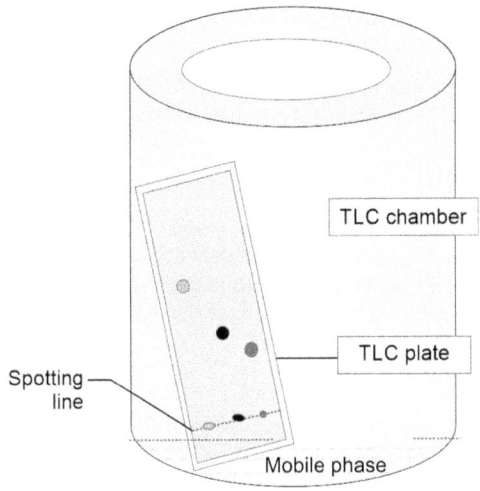

Figure 14.5: Separation of compounds by thin layer chromatography.

THIN LAYER CHROMATOGRAPHY (TLC) AND APPLICATIONS

Separation of compounds on a thin layer is similar in many ways to paper chromatography. Just like other chromatography processes, this one consists of a **mobile phase** and a **stationary phase.** The stationary phase is a thin layer of adsorbent material, such as aluminum oxide, silica gel, or cellulose. This layer is applied to plastic, glass, or aluminum foil sheets called an inert substrate **(Figure 14.5).** The mobile phase is a suitable liquid solvent or mixture of solvents.

Principle

TLC is based on the chromatography principle where components of the mixture are separated between a fixed stationary phase and a liquid mobile phase by differential affinities between the two phases. The components having more affinity for stationary phase travel slower while components with less affinity for stationary phase travel faster. The separated components appear as spots on the plate and the retention factor (Rf) of each component is assessed.

Procedure

The stationary phase that is applied to the plate is made to dry and stabilize. Ready-made TLC plates are preferred.
- To apply sample spots, thin marks are made at the bottom of the plate with the help of a pencil.
- Apply sample solutions to the marked spots.
- Pour the mobile phase into the TLC chamber.
- The plate is then immersed in the TLC chamber such that the sample spots are well above the level of the mobile phase and close it with a lid.
- Allow sufficient time for the separation and development of spots. Then remove the plates and allow them to dry. The sample spots can be observed under UV light chamber or any other methods as recommended for the said sample.

Applications of TLC

- TLC can be used to analyze; pesticides, steroids, alkaloids, lipids, nucleotides, glycosides, carbohydrates, and fatty acids.
- TLC is widely used by many industries and research fields, including pharmaceuticals, clinical testing, environmental toxicology, food, water and pesticide analysis, and cosmetics. Typical applications of TLC include:
  - Analysis of drug residues and antibiotics in food and environmental samples
  - Identification and quantification of colors, ingredients, preservatives, and sweetening agents in food and cosmetic products

- Quality control and purity testing of pharmaceutical formulations
- For separation of phospholipids.
- For determination of lecithin/sphingomyelin ratio in cases of respiratory distress syndrome
- It is used for identification of toxic drugs in cases of poisoning.

QUESTIONS

1. Define chromatography and write various types of chromatography.
2. Write the principle of paper chromatography.
3. Write the applications of paper chromatographic technique.
4. Write the applications of thin layer chromatographic technique.

EXPERIMENT 15

Arterial Blood Gas (ABG) Analyzer

COMPETENCY	LEARNING OBJECTIVES
BI11.16 Observe the use of commonly used equipments/techniques in biochemistry laboratory including: pH meter, paper chromatography, protein electrophoresis, TLC, PAGE, electrolyte analysis by ISE, ABG analyzer, ELISA, immunodiffusion, autoanalyser, quality control and DNA isolation from blood tissue. **BI11.19** Outline the basic principles involved in the functioning of instruments commonly used in a biochemistry laboratory and their applications.	1. Describe the principle and components of ABG analyzer. 2. Describe blood sample collection for ABG analysis. 3. Describe use of ABG analyzer with its clinical significance. 4. Describe clinical cases based on acid base imbalance.

INTRODUCTION

The assessment of acid-base status is usually done by **arterial blood gas (ABG) analyzer (Figure 15.1)** which measures **pH, pCO$_2$,** and **pO$_2$** directly by means of electrodes. Arterial blood gas analysis is a common investigation in **emergency** departments and **intensive care** units for monitoring patients with **acute respiratory failure.**

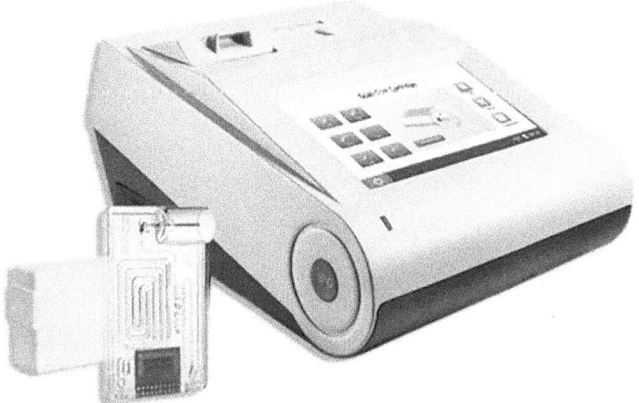

Figure 15.1: Arterial blood gas (ABG) analyzer.

PRINCIPLE AND COMPONENTS OF ABG ANALYZER

Principle

It is based on the principle of potentiometry. Potentiometry is the method to find the concentration of solute in a given solution by measuring the potential between two electrodes. ABG analyzer measures pH, pCO_2, and pO_2 directly by means of electrodes.

Components of ABG Analyzer

- **Sample probe:** For presenting the blood specimen
- **Reference electrodes:** For measuring the potential difference
- **Gas electrodes:** For measuring pCO_2, and pO_2 concentrations
- **Pump:** For pumping the waste after the specimen is analyzed
- **Valve:** To monitor the flow of specimen
- Central processing unit (CPU)
- Display unit

BLOOD SAMPLE COLLECTION: FOR ABG ANALYSIS

An arterial blood sample is collected from radial artery by using a needle and syringe to puncture an artery. These syringes are pre-heparinized and handled to minimize air exposure that will alter the blood gas values.

Sampling errors: Inappropriate collection and handling of arterial blood specimens can produce incorrect results. Reasons for an inaccurate blood result include:
- Presence of air in the sample
- Collection of venous rather than arterial blood
- An improper quantity of heparin in the syringe, or improper mixing after blood is drawn.
- A delay in specimen transportation

USE OF ABG ANALYZER AND CLINICAL SIGNIFICANCE

Arterial blood gas analyzer measures the amounts of arterial gases, which includes the following:
- **Oxygen content (O_2CT):** This measures the amount of oxygen in blood.
- **Oxygen saturation (SaO_2):** This measures how much hemoglobin in blood is carrying oxygen.
- **Partial pressure of oxygen (pO_2):** This measure the pressure of oxygen dissolved in blood.
- **Partial pressure of carbon dioxide (pCO_2):** This measures the amount of carbon dioxide in blood.
- **pH:** This measures blood pH level.
- **Bicarbonate (HCO_3):** This is calculated using the measured values of pH and PCO_2.

Normal Adult Values of Various Parameters of ABG

- **pH:** 7.35–7.45
- **pO_2:** 80–100 mm Hg
- **pCO_2:** 35–45 mm Hg
- **HCO_3^-:** 22–26 mEq/L
- **Oxygen saturation (SaO_2):** 95–100%

Clinical Significance

An arterial blood gas analysis can help in the assessment of a patient's **gas exchange, ventilatory control,** and **acid base balance** and to diagnose acid base disorders (**Figure 15.2**). **Table 15.1** summarizes the clinical causes of acid-base disorders. The test also determines whether body compensates for the acid base imbalance. Compensatory responses are given in **Table 15.2**.

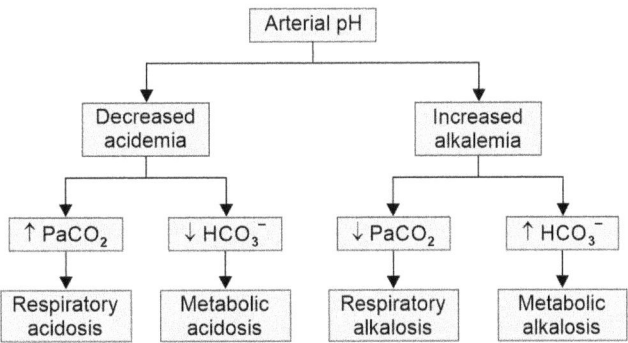

Figure 15.2: Analysis of acid base disorders.

Table 15.1: Acid-base disorders and their clinical causes.

Acid-base disorders	Clinical causes
Metabolic acidosis	• Diabetes mellitus (Ketoacidosis) • Lactic acidosis • Therapeutic administration of HCL • Renal failure • Severe diarrhea • Renal tubular acidosis due to loss of HCO_3^- ions
Respiratory acidosis	• Chronic obstructive pulmonary disease (COPD), asthma, emphysema, and pneumonia • Cardiac arrest, severe hypoxia • Administration of respiratory depressant toxic drugs, e.g., morphine
Metabolic alkalosis	• Loss of gastric juice along with H⁺ ions • Therapeutic administration of alkali
Respiratory alkalosis	• Hyperventilation (anxiety, fever) • Hot baths • High altitudes • Working at high temperature • Salicylate poisoning

Table 15.2: Acid base disorders with their compensatory response.

Disorder	pH	Primary disturbance	Compensatory response
Metabolic acidosis	↓	↓ (HCO_3^-)	↓ pCO_2
Metabolic alkalosis	↑	↑ (HCO_3^-)	↑ pCO_2
Respiratory acidosis	↓	↑ pCO_2	↑ (HCO_3^-)
Respiratory alkalosis	↑	↓ pCO_2	↓ (HCO_3^-)

Clinical Cases Based on Acid Base Imbalance

❖ A young man with a history of dyspepsia and excessive alcohol intake who gives a history of vomiting. Blood gas results are:
- pH = 7.5 (alkalosis);
- HCO_3^- = 47 mEq/L (Normal 22–26 mEq/L) (metabolic alkalosis due to loss of H⁺ from gut).
- PCO_2 = 55 mm Hg (Normal 35–45 mm Hg) (respiratory acidosis, signifying compensation).

❖ A patient who has had an acute asthmatic attack. Blood gas results are:
- pH = 7.6 (alkalosis);
- pCO_2 = 20 mm Hg (Normal 35–45 mm Hg) (respiratory alkalosis);
- HCO_3^- = 22 mEq/L (Normal 22–26 mEq/L) (not low, hence uncompensated); therefore uncompensated respiratory alkalosis.

❖ A patient with chronic bronchitis. Blood gas results are:
  - pH = 7.356 (normal, so there is either no acid-base disturbance or a fully compensated one);
  - PCO_2 = 70 mm Hg (Normal 35-45 mm Hg) (respiratory acidosis); HCO_3^- = 40 mEq/L (Normal 22-26 mEq/L) (metabolic alkalosis)

In view of the history, it will most likely to be a fully compensated respiratory acidosis. The other possibility is a fully compensated metabolic alkalosis.

QUESTIONS

1. Write principle of ABG analyzer.
2. What are the components of ABG analyzer?
3. Write normal adults values of various parameter of ABG.
4. Write use of ABG analyzer.
5. Write clinical application of ABG analyzer.

EXPERIMENT 16

Composition of CSF

COMPETENCY	LEARNING OBJECTIVES
BI11.15 Describe and discuss the composition of CSF.	1. Describe formation, composition, functions of CSF. 2. Describe collection of CSF sample. 3. Describe examination of CSF and interpret findings of CSF glucose and protein in pathological conditions.

INTRODUCTION

Cerebrospinal fluid (CSF) is a clear, colorless fluid found in and around the brain and spinal cord. It protects the brain and spinal cord by acting like a liquid cushion. Inside the skull, the cerebrospinal fluid is contained within the subarachnoid space and the central canal of the spinal cord.

FORMATION, COMPOSITION, FUNCTIONS OF CEREBROSPINAL FLUID (CSF)

Formation of CSF

- CSF is formed by two different processes, namely **active secretion** and **ultrafiltration:**
    1. **Active secretion** is brought about by **choroid plexus** located in the ventricles (hollow spaces within the brain) of the brain.
    2. **Ultrafiltration** is brought about by blood vessels that are present in ventricular regions
- The total volume of CSF in adults is about **150 mL**. It is constantly produced and absorbed through the subarachnoid villi into the venous system to keep volume constant.
- Around 500 mL of CSF is produced each day (around 0.3 mL/min). Total amount of CSF is replaced every 6 to 8 hours.
- If absorption is impaired (as after meningeal inflammation, bacterial meningitis, or subarachnoid hemorrhage) CNS pressure and CSF volume both raise, this is called a **communicating hydrocephalus**.
- The meninges are the three membranes (the dura, arachnoid, and pia) that covering the brain and spinal cord.

Composition of CSF

Cerebrospinal fluid (CSF) is a clear, watery fluid. It is an ultrafiltrate of blood plasma. Composition of CSF is qualitatively similar to composition of blood plasma **(Table 16.1)**. However quantitatively it differs from plasma.

- CSF contains chiefly proteins, glucose, lactate, ammonia, glutamine, LDH, adenosine deaminase, creatinine, urea and electrolytes, such as sodium (Na^+), potassium (K^+), calcium (Ca^{++}), magnesium (Mg^+), and chloride (Cl^-).
- Compared with plasma, CSF has less protein, glucose, potassium, and calcium and more sodium and chloride.

Infection or the presence of blood in the CSF alters its composition. This provides the basis for biochemical analysis of CSF in the diagnosis of **subarachnoid hemorrhage (SAH)** and **meningitis.**

Table 16.1: Composition and characteristics of normal CSF.

Parameters	Normal values
Total volume	150 mL
Color	Colorless
Transparency	Clear like water
Osmolarity	290 to 295 mOsm/L
Specific gravity	1.006 to 1.008
pH	7.7
Cell count	0 to 5 WBCs per cubic millimeter (mm^3)
Sodium	138 to 150 mEq/L
Potassium	2.7 to 3.9 mEq/L
Chloride	120 to 130 mEq/L
Calcium	2.0 to 2.5 mEq/L (4 to 5 mg/L)
Magnesium	2.0 to 2.5 mEq/L (2.4 to 3.1 mg/L)
Glucose	40 to 80 mg/dL
Proteins	15 to 45 mg/dL

FUNCTIONS OF CSF

CSF has several functions in the nervous system. For example it:
- Provides mechanical support to the brain.
- Protects the brain and spinal cord from trauma. It acts as a shock absorber, cushioning the brain against the skull.
- Supplies nutrients to nervous system tissue.
- Removes waste products from cerebral metabolism.
- Protects the brain during blood pressure fluctuations.
- Regulates the chemical environment of the central nervous system and it is a vehicle for intracerebral transport.

Collection of CSF

- A sample of the CSF is obtained through a **lumbar puncture (LP)**, also called spinal tap, in which the **spinal needle** is inserted in the subarachnoid space between lumbar vertebrae L3 and L4 or L4 and L5. The patient is placed so as to facilitate access **(Figure 16.1)**.
- The typical procedure involves laying on side in a fetal position. The neck is bent so the chin is close to the chest and both knees are drawn up toward the chest. After the fluid is collected and the needle is removed, the patient is asked to lie on his/her back or stomach for a few hours after the procedure to prevent a spinal headache.
- Universal sterile screw capped container without any additive is used to collect CSF samples **(Figure 16. 2)**. Up to 20 mL of CSF can be safely removed.

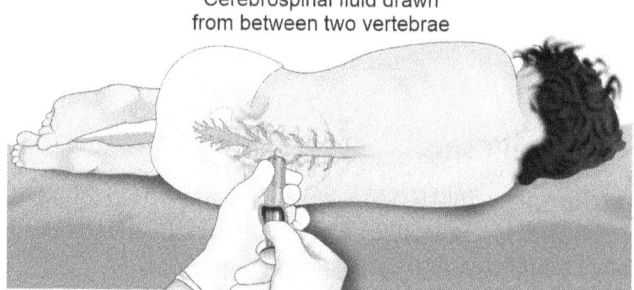
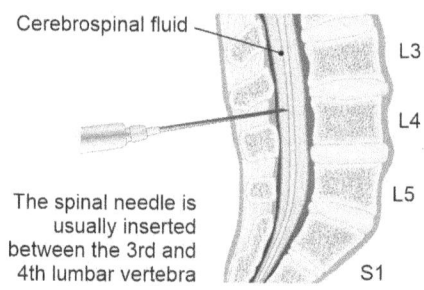

Figure 16.1: Lumber puncture site for CSF sample collection.

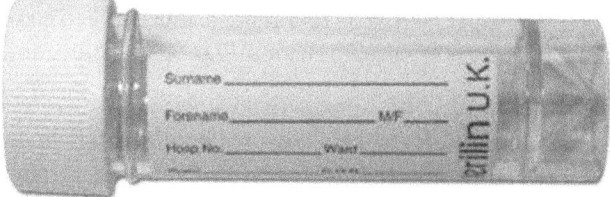

Figure 16.2: Universal sterile screw capped container without any additive to collect CSF samples.

- Sample should be drawn to divide into three containers to carry out three routine investigations:
  - *1st container:* Biochemistry and immunology studies
  - *2nd container:* Microbiological examination
  - *3rd container:* Cytology studies (for cell count and differential)
- Specimens should be delivered to the laboratory as soon as possible and processed quickly to minimize cellular and chemical degradation.

EXAMINATION OF CSF

The examination of the CSF is of great diagnostic aid in differentiating certain neurological conditions, such as:
- Meningeal infection (bacterial meningitis, viral, tuberculous or fungal meningitis). Meningitis refers to inflammation of the meninges which line the CNS.
- Subarachnoid hemorrhage
- CNS malignancies (primary and metastatic)
- Demyelinating diseases, e.g., multiple sclerosis

CSF biochemistry is usually performed in conjunction with microbiology and cytology examination.

Physical Examination of CSF

- Normal CSF is clear and colorless and viscosity is similar to that of water. The viscosity of CSF may increase due to spread of mucin producing adenocarcinoma cells or cryptococcal infection.
- It may appear turbid or cloudy due to increase cell counts (leukocytes) and protein. The presence of bacteria may also cause turbidity of the specimen.
- The color of CSF may be yellow due to presence of bilirubin or brown by methemoglobin. Yellow discoloration of CSF is called xanthochromia.
- A **bright red color** may result from damage to a blood vessel during lumber puncture (traumatic tap), or due to bleeding into the subarachnoid space called **subarachnoid hemorrhage (SAH)**. If CSF is collected in three separate containers, blood staining will be progressively less in the containers if bleeding is due to the lumber puncture itself, whereas all containers would be expected to be bloody if there was a subarachnoid hemorrhage. In subarachnoid hemorrhage, the patient typically complains of a **severe headache** of sudden onset, often associated with **vomiting.**

Biochemical Examination of CSF

Most commonly biochemical constituents estimated in biochemistry lab are **glucose** and **protein**.

CSF Glucose

- Normal range of CSF glucose is 40–80 mg/dL based on plasma glucose. Simultaneous blood glucose assessment is important to have correct interpretation.
- Increased glucose in CSF denotes hyperglycemia and clinically not very significant.
- The decrease in CSF glucose is called **hypoglycorrhachia**. Hypoglycorrhachia may be due to increased metabolism of glucose by cell or microorganism (bacterial, fungal) which is usually observed in infections such as **(Table 16.2)**.
  - Bacterial meningitis
  - Tuberculous meningitis
  - Fungal meningitis
- Viral meningitis does not often cause low glucose levels in the CSF. It is often normal or slightly elevated.

CSF Protein

The spinal fluid normally contains very little protein since serum proteins are large molecules that do not cross the blood-brain barrier. Most of the protein that is normally present is **albumin**. More than 80% of the CSF protein content is derived from blood plasma.

CSF total protein determination test may be helpful in diagnosing tumors, infective polyneuritis (inflammation of nerve cells), vasculitis (inflammation of the blood vessels), blood in the CSF, and trauma.

- ❖ Normal range of CSF protein is 15–45 mg/dL. CSF protein concentration may rise due to two factors:
    1. Either an increased permeability of the blood brain barrier allowing more protein and higher molecular weight proteins to enter the CSF or
    2. Proteins may be synthesized within the cerebrospinal canal by inflammatory or other invading cells.
- ❖ The increase in CSF proteins is observed in following conditions **(Table 16.2)**
- ❖ Meningitis (bacterial, fungal, tuberculous). In viral meningitis, protein level may be normal or elevated.
- ❖ Hemorrhage (subarachnoid, intracerebral)
- ❖ Mechanical obstruction (tumor, abscess, herniated disk)
- ❖ Increased immunoglobulin synthesis (multiple sclerosis)

Table: 16.2: CSF parameters in normal and some common disorders.

Parameters	Normal	Viral meningitis	Bacterial meningitis	Tuberculous meningitis	Fungal meningitis	Subarachnoid hemorrhage
Appearance	Clear	Clear	Turbid	Clear/Turbid (cobweb coagulum)	Turbid	Grossly bloody, xanthochromic or clear
White blood cells	0 to 5 WBCs per cubic millimeter (mm^3)	Increased (lymphocytes)	Increased (polymorphonuclear leukocytes)	Increased (lymphocytes)	Increased (lymphocytes)	Increased due to bleeding
Glucose	2/3rd of plasma glucose	Normal/Increased	Marked decreased	Decreased	Decreased	Normal
Proteins	15–45 mg/dL	No change/mild elevation	Marked elevation	Elevation	Elevation	Elevated

QUESTIONS

1. What is CSF?
2. What are functions of CSF?
3. Write composition and characteristics of normal CSF.
4. How the CSF sample is collected for analysis?
5. Write different normal and abnormal physical characteristics of CSF.
6. What is the normal range of protein in CSF and write its clinical significance?
7. What is the normal range of glucose in CSF and write its clinical significance?

SECTION B
Qualitative Experiments DOAP/SGD

Section Outline

Experiment 17: Physical and Chemical Components of Normal Urine and Analysis of Normal Urine
Experiment 18: Physical and Chemical Components and Analysis of Abnormal Urine and Interpretation
Experiment 19: Screening of Urine for Inborn Errors and Use of Paper Chromatography

EXPERIMENT 17

Physical and Chemical Components of Normal Urine and Analysis of Normal Urine

COMPETENCY		LEARNING OBJECTIVES
BI11.3	Describe the chemical components of normal urine.	1. Describe the physical and chemical components of normal urine.
BI11.4	Perform urine analysis to estimate and determine normal and abnormal constituents.	2. Perform tests for the normal constituents of urine.

INTRODUCTION

Urine is an excretory product formed by the kidneys. Its analysis is important in evaluating kidney functions as well as diagnosis of many diseases.

PHYSICAL AND CHEMICAL COMPONENTS OF NORMAL URINE

Urine is normally composed of:
- About 99% water
- About **1% solids** which are:
  - **Inorganic salts:** Inorganic sulfates, phosphates and chlorides of Na/K, salts of ammonia
  - Nitrogenous organic compounds, such as urea, uric acids, creatinine, hippuric acid
  - Organic sulfur containing compounds, such as ethereal sulfates.

Physical Characteristics

- **Volume:** The daily output of urine in adult is 1000 to 2000 mL with an average of **1,500 mL/day.** The quantity normally depends on the water intake, the external temperature, the diet and the mental and physical state, cardiovascular and renal function.
- **Color:** Normal urine is pale yellow or amber color due to pigment urobilin. Variation in color may be physiological or pathological. Darkening from the normal pale yellow color indicates more concentrated urine or presence of another pigment, such as hemoglobin (hematuria) and myoglobin (rhabdomyolysis) in urine produce a reddish coloration.
- **Odor:** Normally aromatic but turns ammonical on standing due to urea splitting organisms, liberating ammonia. Foul smell indicates bacterial infection.

- ❖ **Appearance:** Freshly voided urine is clear and transparent but becomes turbid on standing due to precipitation of phosphates and urates. Turbidity in a fresh sample may indicate infection but also may be due to fat particles in an individual with nephrotic syndrome.
- ❖ **pH:** The urine is normally acidic with a pH of about 6.0 (range 4.8-7.5) when fresh and becomes alkaline on standing due to conversion to ammonia. Very often urine excreted after ingestion of vegetarian diet is alkaline and that excreted after intake of non-vegetarian diet is acidic.
- ❖ **Specific gravity:** The specific gravity indicates the concentrating ability of the kidney. It normally varies from **1.012 to 1.024**. It can vary widely depending on diet, fluid intake and renal function. If renal function is impaired, the quantity of eliminated urine will be very less. In this condition, increased specific gravity may be seen. It is measured using an instrument called urinometer **(Figure 17.1)**. It is calibrated at **15°C** with specific gravity of water which is 1. It consists of a thin stem graduated from 1,000-1,060 corresponding to specific gravities of 1.00-1.06 values. As it is calibrated at 15°C, temperature correction has to be applied as follows:
  - For every 6°C rise in room temperature, add 0.001 to the observed specific gravity.
  - For every 6°C fall in room temperature, subtract 0.001 from the observed specific gravity.

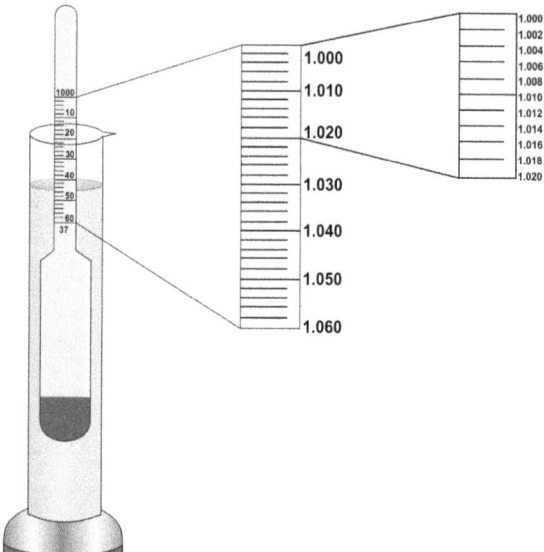

Figure 17.1: Measurement of specific gravity by urinometer.

- ❖ **Total solids:** Total dissolved solids in urine constitute between 25 to 50 g/L. Urinary solids are primarily made up of organic matter. The concentration of solids in urine can be measured by multiplying last 2 digits of specific gravity with 2.66 (Long's coefficient).

Chemical Constituents

Normal urine contains both **organic** and **inorganic** constituents.

Inorganic Constituents

The urine contains inorganic constituents, such as cations like Na^+, K^+, Ca^{2+}, and Mg^{2+} which are excreted as salts in association with anions like SO_4^{2-}, PO_4^{2-}, etc.
- ❖ **Chlorides:** Chlorides are excreted mainly in the form of sodium chloride. The amount of sodium chloride excreted varies between 5 to 25 grams per day depending upon diet.
- ❖ **Sulfates:** Sulfate is derived from catabolism of sulfur containing amino acids (cystine, cysteine, and methionine). The sulfur is metabolized and excreted in two forms—inorganic sulfates and organic ethereal sulfates.
- ❖ **Calcium:** Under normal dietary intake, urinary excretion of calcium is 100-200 mg/day.
- ❖ **Phosphates:** The phosphate is derived chiefly from the metabolism of phosphorus containing foodstuffs and tissue components, such as phosphoproteins, nucleoproteins, nucleotides and phospholipids. The quantity excreted is extremely variable as it depends on the nature of the diet. Phosphorus is excreted in urine largely as inorganic phosphate and to small extent in organic form (<4% of total).
- ❖ **Ammonia:** Urinary ammonia is derived from glutamine and other amino acids in kidney. Under normal dietary conditions, an adult excretes 0.5-1 gram of ammonia daily.

Organic Constituents

- ❖ **Urea:** It is the principle end product of protein (amino acid) metabolism. About 20 to 6 grams of urea is excreted per day. The amount excreted depends on protein intake.

EXPERIMENT 17: Physical and Chemical Components of Normal Urine and Analysis of Normal Urine

- ❖ **Creatinine:** Creatinine is formed during muscle metabolism from creatine phosphate. It is anhydride of creatine. The amount of creatinine excreted in urine is 1–2 g/day. It is purely endogenous and does not depend on the dietary intake of proteins. The amount of creatinine excreted in urine is dependent on muscle mass.
- ❖ **Uric acid:** It is the end product of purine nucleotide catabolism. The quantity of uric acid excreted in urine varies from 0.5 to 1 g/day. The amount of uric acid excretion is dependent on purine intake.
- ❖ **Hippuric acid:** Hippuric acid represents a detoxication product of benzoic acid with glycine. Benzoic acid is present in many fruits, vegetables and also as food preservatives. The amount of hippuric acid excreted per day in urine varies between 0.1 to 1 g/day with average of about 0.7 grams per day.
- ❖ **Ethereal sulfates:** about 100 mg of organic sulfate is excreted per day. They consist of sodium and potassium salts of sulfuric acid esters of phenols, such as indoxyl, skatoxyl, phenol and cresol. These are detoxication compounds of phenols and are found in liver. Indoxyl and skatoxyl sulfates are formed by putrefactive decomposition of tryptophan in the intestine.
- ❖ **Urobilinogen:** It is colorless compound formed during the metabolism of heme. Normally, trace amount (0.4 mg/day) of urobilinogen is excreted through urine. The amount of urobilinogen present in urine depends on the amount of bilirubin from liver entering the intestine.
  - An increase in urobilinogen in urine is found in hemolytic jaundice due to excess production of bilirubin.
  - In hepatitis, the urobilinogen in urine may be normal or decreased.
  - In post-hepatic obstructive jaundice, due to the complete or almost complete biliary obstruction, no urobilinogen is found in urine because bilirubin is unable to enter the intestine.

TESTS FOR THE NORMAL CONSTITUENTS OF URINE

Tests for normal inorganic constituents of urine are given in **Table 17.1** and tests for normal organic constituents of urine are given in **Table 17.2**.

Table 17.1: Tests for normal inorganic constituents of urine.

Test	Observation	Inference
Test for chloride To 2 mL of urine, add 0.5 mL of conc. nitric acid and 2 mL of 3% silver nitrate	Curdy white precipitate	Chloride is precipitated as silver chloride with $AgNO_3$, in the presence of HNO_3
Test for calcium To 5 mL urine, add 5 drops of 1% acetic acid and 5 mL of 2% Potassium oxalate	Trace amount of white Precipitate	Calcium is precipitated as calcium oxalate
Test for inorganic phosphate To 5 mL urine, add 5 drops of conc. HNO_3, and a pinch of ammonium molybdate. Warm and observe.	Canary yellow color or precipitate (a green color indicates nitric acid is Insufficient).	Inorganic phosphate is precipitated as canary Yellow ammonium phosphomolybdate
Test for inorganic sulfate To 2 mL urine, add 1 mL conc. HCl and 2 mL of 10% $BaCl_2$. Mix	White precipitate is formed.	Sulfate is precipitated as barium sulfate With barium chloride
Test for ammonia To 5 mL urine, add 1–2 mL of 2% Na_2Co_3. Boil the solution, hold a piece of moistened red litmus paper at the mouth of the test tube	Red litmus turns blue	Ammonia liberated turns red litmus paper to blue

Table 17.2: Tests for normal organic constituents of urine.

Sl. No.	Test	Observation	Inference
1.	**Tests for urea:** **Specific urease test** 3 ml urine + a drop of phenolphthalein + a pinch urease powder. Shake the contents of the tube and allow to stand for 10 minutes	Intense pink color after 10 minutes	Urea is hydrolyzed by urease to form $(NH_4)_2CO_3$ which makes the solution alkaline. Hence, phenolphthalein turns pink
	Hypobromite test 3 mL urine + few drops of sodium hypobromite solution (freshly prepared). This test is unstable	Effervescence which disappears quickly	Urea is decomposed by hypobromite to release nitrogen gas
2.	**Test for creatinine:** **Jaffe's Test** 3 mL saturated picric acid solution + 3 mL 5% NaOH solution. Mix and add 2 mL urine	Orange red color	Creatinine reacts with picric acid in alkaline medium to form orange red colored creatinine picrate.
3.	**Test for uric acid:** Make urine alkaline by adding 1 mL of 2% sodium carbonates to 3 mL urine in a test tube and use alkaline urine for the following tests. (Uric acid acts as reducing agent in alkaline medium). **i. Schiff's test** Add 2–3 drops of $AgNO_3$ on filter paper. Add 5–6 drops of urine (alkaline). Warm gently, if necessary	Greyish /Black spot develops	In alkaline medium uric acid reduces $AgNO_3$ to metallic silver.
	ii. Benedict's uric acid test 3 mL urine (alkaline) + 0.5 mL of Benedict's uric acid reagent and mix the content by shaking the tube	Blue color	Uric acid reduces phosphotungstic acid, present in Benedict's uric acid reagent, to blue colored tungstate salt
4.	**Test for hippuric acid:** 3 mL urine + 1 mL of 5% NaOH + dilute $FeCl_3$ solution drop by drop	Cream-colored precipitate	Formation of cream colored ferric hippurate.
5.	**Test for ethereal sulfate:** To 3 mL urine, add 1 mL conc. HCl and 2 mL of 10% BaCl2. Mix and filter. Boil for 2 minutes and cool at room temperature.	A trace turbidity is formed due to presence of organic SO_4	Ethereal sulfates are dissociated on boiling with conc. HCL to liberate inorganic sulfates, which form white precipitate of barium sulfate
6.	**Test for urobilinogen:** **Ehrlich's aldehyde test** 5 mL urine + 5 mL Ehrlich's reagent. Mix, wait for 10 minutes then add 10 mL saturated sodium acetate.	Pinkish-color obtained	Ehrlich's reagent (2% para-Dimethylaminobenzaldehyde in 20% HCl) reacts with urobilinogen to from a pinkish-colored compound

EXPERIMENT 17: Physical and Chemical Components of Normal Urine and Analysis of Normal Urine

RESULTS

Physical Characteristics

Characteristics: **Observations**
1. Volume
2. Color
3. Appearance
4. Odor
5. pH
6. Specific gravity
   Room temperature
   Calibration temperature
   Temperature difference
   Observed specific gravity
   Therefore, corrected specific gravity
   $= \text{Observed sp. gr.} + \dfrac{(0.001 \times \text{Temp. diff.})}{3}$
7. Total solids
   = Last two digits of sp. gr. x 2.66 =...............................g/lit.

Chemical Components Present in Normal Urine

- Inorganic...
- Organic..

ASSESSMENT QUESTION

Q. Urine analysis.
Perform tests for the normal constituents of urine in the given sample.

VIVA QUESTIONS

1. Which are the normal constituents of urine?
2. What is the normal urine volume excreted per day?
3. Why normal urine having pale yellow color?
4. What are the common causes of turbidity seen in a fresh urine sample?
5. Why does a normal appearing urine sample sometimes become turbid on standing?
6. Which instrument is used to measures the specific gravity of urine?
7. What is the normal specific gravity of urine?
8. Name the tests to perform for urea.
9. What is hippuric acid?
10. What is urobilinogen? In which abnormal conditions it is excreted in large amount?

EXPERIMENT 18

Physical and Chemical Components and Analysis of Abnormal Urine and Interpretation

COMPETENCY	LEARNING OBJECTIVES
BI11.4 Perform urine analysis to estimate and determine normal and abnormal constituents. **BI11.20** Identify abnormal constituents in urine, interpret the findings and correlate these with pathological states.	1. Describe and determine the physical parameters and chemical constituents of abnormal urine. 2. Perform analysis of abnormal of urine and interpret the results and correlate these with pathological states.

INTRODUCTION

Routine urine examination is usually the first test undertaken to assess the renal function and very often it gives some important information, such as **proteinuria, hematuria** to do further renal investigation. Its analysis, therefore, is important in evaluating kidney function. It may reveal the disease anywhere in the urinary tract. The standard urine analysis includes:
- Physical examination
- Chemical examination
- Microscopic examination of urine

PHYSICAL PARAMETERS AND CHEMICAL COMPONENTS OF ABNORMAL URINE

Physical Parameters

Volume: The daily output of urine in adult is 1000 to 2000 mL with an average of **1,500 mL/day.**
- An increase in urine output is called **polyuria** (> 2000 mL/day).
- It is observed in diabetes mellitus, diabetes insipidus, excess water intake and intake of diuretics, such as caffeine, alcohol, etc.
- Decrease in urine output is called **Oliguria** (< 500 mL/day)
- It is observed in fluid deprivation, excess fluid loss as in hemorrhage, neurogenic shock, dehydration, acute glomerulonephritis and obstruction in the urinary tract.
- A total suppression of urine formation is called **anuria:** (Complete absence of urine output).
  It is observed in shock and renal failure.

Appearance: Clear when fresh
- Turbidity in urine implies the presence of pus or bacteria
- Turbidity on standing is due to precipitation of phosphates
- Milky appearance of urine is due to the presence of fat droplets (chyluria)

Color: Normal urine is pale yellow or amber color
- Dark yellow in high fever (due to concentrated urine) and jaundice
- Smoky red due to the presence of RBCs
- Yellowish brown or greenish due to the presence of bilirubin in case of obstructive jaundice.
- Dark brown/black upon standing in alkaptonuria

Odor: Normal urine has aromatic odor.
- Ammonical on standing due to urea splitting organisms
- Fruity odor is due to the presence of acetone in diabetic ketoacidosis
- Mousy odor in Phenylketonuria
- Maple syrup odor in congenital Maples syrup urine disease
- Boiled cabbage odor in tyrosinemia.

pH: Variations of urinary pH occur due to acid-base disturbances.
- **Alkaline urine is voided in:** Metabolic alkalosis in severe vomiting, respiratory alkalosis in hyperventilation
- Acidic urine is voided in in fever, diabetic ketoacidosis.

Specific gravity: Normal range is 1.012 to 1.024.
- Presence of abnormal constituents, such as glucose or proteins increase specific gravity
- In diabetes insipidus low specific gravity is observed due to polyuria.
- Increase in specific gravity is observed in acute nephritis and fever when concentrated urine is excreted.
- Fat decreases specific gravity as observed in chyluria.

Chemical Constituents

The abnormal constituents which are routinely analyzed in urine are **protein (albumin, Bence-Jones protein), blood, glucose, ketone bodies, bile salts** and **bile pigment.** The abnormal constituents that appear in different disease conditions are listed in **Table 18.1.**

- **Protein:** When glomeruli are damaged or diseased, they become more permeable and plasma proteins appear in urine. Presence of detectable amount of protein in urine is known as **proteinuria.** The smaller molecules of albumin pass through damaged glomeruli more readily than the heavier globulin and so most commonly albumin is seen in urine (**albuminuria**) and is characteristic of kidney disease, such as nephrotic syndrome, glomerulonephritis, diabetic nephropathy, hypertensive nephropathy, renal failure as well as congestive heart failure.
- **Glucose:** Presence of glucose in urine is called as **glycosuria**. This usually occurs in hyperglycemia. **Hyperglycemic glucosuria** is usually seen when plasma glucose rises above the renal threshold of 180 mg/dL as in **diabetes mellitus**. However, glycosuria is not always due to diabetes. **Renal glucosuria** (in pregnancy) presence of glucose in urine even at normal plasma concentrations is due to impaired reabsorption of glucose in the proximal tubule\which is unrelated to diabetes.
- **Ketones bodies (β-hydroxybutyrate, acetoacetate** and **acetone):** Excretion of ketone bodies in urine is called **ketonuria.** Ketone bodies do not appear in urine because ketone bodies which are produced normally in liver are completely oxidized in tissues. If fats are metabolized excessively as in **diabetes** (diabetic ketoacidosis), in **alcoholism** (alcoholic ketoacidosis) or in **starvation**, there will be overproduction of ketone bodies. The tissues are unable to oxidize the excessive amount ketone bodies which are excreted through urine.
- **Blood:** The presence of blood in the urine is called **hematuria** and is seen in diseases of kidney or urinary tract, such as **acute glomerulonephritis, renal stones** or **urinary tract infections. Hemoglobinuria** refers to the presence of hemoglobin in urine, which occurs due to intravascular hemolysis, e.g., **malaria, severe burns, hemolytic jaundice** and **enteric fever.**
- **Bile salts:** Normally bile salts are not excreted in urine and are absent in the urine. Bile salts appear in the urine when there is an obstruction to the biliary tract (cholestasis). In obstructive jaundice, they appear in urine. Hay's sulfur test is done to detect the presence of bile salts. Bile salts lower the surface tension of liquids and so when sulfur powder is sprinkled on urine it sinks down. When bile salts are absent, sulfur will remain (float) on the surface.
- **Bile pigment (Bilirubin):** The detectable amount of bilirubin is not found in the urine. Breakdown of hemoglobin leads to bilirubin formation, which goes to the liver. From the liver excreted into the bile. Bilirubin is a yellowish

Table 18.1: The abnormal constituents that appear in different disease conditions.

Constituent	Clinical significance	Abnormal conditions
Protein	**Glomerular proteinuria** refers to the presence of albumin in urine due to a loss of integrity of the glomerular basement membrane	Nephrotic syndrome, acute glomerulonephritis, diabetic nephropathy, etc.
	Overflow proteinuria is due to the presence of abnormally high levels of low molecular weight proteins in the plasma that are filtered by the glomerulus and thus appear in the urine	Multiple myeloma (light chains of immunoglobulins appear in urine, resulting in Bence-Jones proteinuria)
	Tubular proteinuria refers to the presence of low molecular weight proteins (such as β_2 microglobulin) in urine, due to impaired reabsorption of these proteins by the proximal tubule	Fanconi's syndrome, nephrotoxicity due to amino glycoside antibiotics, heavy metals, etc.
	Postrenal proteinuria refers to the presence of proteins in urine derived from the urinary tract	Urinary tract infection (UTI) resulting in inflammatory exudates in urine
Glucose	**Hyperglycemic glucosuria:** Presence of glucose in urine is usually seen when plasma glucose rises above the renal threshold of 180 mg/dL	Uncontrolled diabetes mellitus
	Renal glucosuria: Presence of glucose in urine due to impaired reabsorption of glucose in the proximal tubule	Fanconi's syndrome and inherited defects in the sodium glucose transporter-2 (SGLT-2)
Ketone bodies	Detectable levels in urine (ketonuria) are seen in conditions characterized by increased ketogenesis	Diabetic ketoacidosis and starvation ketoacidosis
Blood	**Hematuria** refers to the presence of red blood cells in urine, due to bleeding into the urinary tract	Renal stones or urinary tract infections
	Hemoglobinuria refers to the presence of hemoglobin in urine, which occurs due to intravascular hemolysis	Incompatible blood transfusions, malaria, etc.
Bile salts and bile pigments	Presence of these in urine is associated with obstruction of the biliary tract	Gall stone or carcinoma of the head of pancreas obstructing the common bile duct

pigment that gives dark yellow or orange color to urine excreted in the urine. It is the conjugated bilirubin, i.e., excreted from the kidneys and appears in the urine. Conjugated bilirubin is water-soluble so it will appear in the urine. Unconjugated bilirubin cannot pass the glomerular filtration, so it is not present in the urine. Excretion of bilirubin is seen in **obstructive jaundice** and **not in hemolytic jaundice** unless there is liver damage. Urine bilirubin is the early sign of **hepatocellular disease** and **intra- or extrahepatic biliary obstruction**.

Microscopic Examination

Microscopic examination of the centrifuged urinary sediment is done to detect cells, such as RBC, WBC, pus cells, crystals, such as calcium phosphate, calcium oxalate, amorphous phosphates, etc., casts, e.g., hyaline casts, granular casts, red blood casts, etc.

Presence of crystals in the urine may be a clue to the diagnosis of a specific type of **renal calculus**. Various components are observed on microscopic examination of urine in renal disease.

ANALYSIS OF ABNORMAL OF URINE AND INTERPRETATION

Most of the physical and chemical parameters can now be estimated semi quantitatively at the bedside using **disposable "dipstick" strips**. Dipsticks are plastic strips on which specific chemicals are impregnated. When the portion of the strip that contains the chemicals is dipped into the sample of urine, they react with specific constituents of urine to produce a color change that is proportional to the concentration of that substance in the sample of urine. Tests for abnormal constituents of urine are given in **Table 18.2**.

Table 18.2: Biochemical tests for abnormal constituents of urine.

Sl. No.	Test	Observation	Inference
1.	**Tests for proteins** **Sulfosalicylic acid test** 3 mL urine + Sulfosalicylic acid drop wise (Bedside test. In emergency, It can be performed when few drops of urine is available)	White precipitate	Protein is present In acidic medium, the proteins acquire a positive charge. The alkaloidal reagent (Sulfosalicylic acid) having negative charge precipitates the protein
	Heller's test In a test tube take 3 mL conc. HNO_3. Add 3 mL urine from side of test tube	White ring at the junction of two layers	Protein is present Concentrated mineral acids HNO_3 cause denaturation of proteins
	Heat coagulation test Take 3/4th test tube full of O.S. heat the upper portion of O.S. Add 1-2 drops of 1% Acetic acid to make it acidic, heat again the upper portion	Turbidity in the upper part due to coagulum which does not dissolve in acetic acid. If precipitate dissolves on adding 1% acetic acid, it is due to phosphates in urine	Protein is present Heat physically denatures the protein. 1% acetic acid dissolves the precipitate formed by acid phosphates in urine. On further heating proteins are irreversibly denatured and precipitated
2	**Test for reducing sugar (glucose)** **Benedict's test** 5 mL Benedict's reagent + 8 drops of urine. Boil for 2 minutes	Green or yellow or orange or red precipitate	Glucose or any reducing sugar is present Glucose reduces alkaline copper sulfate to cuprous oxide which forms colored precipitate. Color of precipitate is suggestive of approximate concentration of glucose in urine: Green (+): 0.5% Yellow (++): 1% Orange (+++): 1.5% Brick Red (++++) : 2% or more It may also be positive in lactosuria, galactosemia, and pentosuria which are identified by other relevant tests
3.	**Test for ketone bodies (acetoacetate and acetone)** **Rothera's test** 5 mL urine + ammonium sulfate powder until saturation + a drop of freshly prepared sodium nitroprusside. Mix and add 2 mL of strong ammonia carefully by the side of the test tube without mixing	A deep purple ring is observed at the junction of two layers β- Hydroxybutyrate does not answer the Rothera's test as it lacks ketone group	Ketone bodies; acetone and acetoacetic acid present Na-nitroprusside reacts with both acetone and acetoacetic acid to produce a purple colored compound
	Gerhard's test for acetoacetate 5 ml urine +10% $FeCl_3$ drop by drop till maximum precipitate of ferric phosphate is formed. Filter and add $FeCl_3$ in excess to filtrate.	Port wine color (mixture of pink and red color)	Acetoacetate is present $FeCl_3$ is added to precipitate the phosphate. After removal of phosphate, $FeCl_3$ reacts with acetoacetate to give Port wine color. For Gerhard's test fresh urine sample should be used, as acetoacetate is quickly decomposed into acetone and CO_2
4.	**Test for blood** **Benzidine test** A pinch of benzidine powder + 3 mL of glacial acetic acid + 3 mL H_2O_2 + 1 mL urine	Blue or green color is formed immediately and disappears	Blood is present Peroxidase in blood decomposes H_2O_2 to liberate nascent oxygen which oxidizes benzidine to bluish green compound

Contd...

Contd...

Sl. No.	Test	Observation	Inference
5.	**Test for bile salts** **Hays sulfur test** Take 3 mL urine in a test tube and sprinkle a pinch of sulfur powder on it. Observe without mixing	Sulfur powder sinks to bottom of the test tube	Bile salts present Bile salts reduce surface tension of liquids Sulfur powder sinks if bile salts are present
	Control 3 mL water + a pinch of sulfur powder on it. Observe without mixing	Sulfur powder floats due to absence of bile salts	When bile salts are absent, sulfur will remain (float) on the surface
6.	**Test for bile pigments** **Fouchet's test** 3 mL urine + pinch of $MgSO_4$ powder or 1 mL of $MgSO_4$ + 2 mL 10% $BaCl_2$. Filter the solution. Unfold the filter paper and to the precipitate on the filter paper add few drops of Fouchet's reagent on the precipitate.	Color changes from yellow to blue-green	Bile pigments present $BaCl_2$ reacts with $MgSO_4$ to form precipitate of $BaSO_4$. Bile pigments are adsorbed on the precipitate. Fouchet's reagent contains TCA and $FeCl_3$ which oxidize bilirubin to green colored biliverdin

URINE REPORT

Name : Date:
Age :
Sex :
Referred by :

Physical Analysis

1. Volume :
2. Appearance :
3. Color :
4. Odor :
5. pH :
6. Specific gravity :
7. Total solid :

Chemical Analysis

1. Sugar : Present/Absent
2. Protein : Present/Absent
3. Ketone bodies : Present/Absent
4. Blood : Present/Absent
5. Bile salts : Present/Absent
6. Bile pigment : Present/Absent

Result: The given urine sample contains _____ and _____ abnormal constituents.

Interpretation: The findings correlate with pathological states: ....

Reporting in charge Checked by

(Student signature) (Doctor signature)

ASSESSMENT QUESTION

Q. Urine analysis.

Analyze the given urine sample, correlate the findings with pathological state and write urine report.

VIVA QUESTIONS

1. What are the abnormal constituents of urine?
2. What is polyuria and in which condition it is occur?
3. What are the common causes of oliguria and anuria?
4. What are the common causes of increase in specific gravity?
5. What is glycosuria? What are its causes?
6. What is the principle of Benedict's test?
7. Why Benedict's test is called as semi-quantitative test?
8. What are the common causes of proteinuria?
9. What are the precautions to be taken in performing Hays sulfur test?
10. What is the principle of benzidine test?
11. Why barium chloride is added in Fouchet's test and why pista green color is produced?
12. Name the ketone bodies. What is their biochemical significance?

EXPERIMENT 19

Screening of Urine for Inborn Errors and Use of Paper Chromatography

COMPETENCY	LEARNING OBJECTIVES
BI11.5 Describe screening of urine for inborn errors and describe the use of paper chromatography.	1. Describe techniques for screening of inborn errors of metabolism (IEM). 2. Describe basic chemical tests for screening of IEM. 3. Describe use of paper chromatography for screening of IEMs.

INTRODUCTION

Inborn errors of metabolism (IEM) are inherited disorders caused by mutations in genes coding for enzymes required in metabolism. The incidence of individual inborn error is very low but collectively it is high.

Most are inherited as autosomal recessive. Some are X-linked and therefore have higher incidence rates in males. Another rare mode of inheritance is linked to mitochondrial DNA.

In most of the disorders, problems arise due to accumulation of abnormal metabolites which are toxic that interfere with normal function, or due to reduced ability to synthesize essential compounds. Early screening of newborn for inborn errors of metabolism is important for detection of treatable disorders before irreversible damage occurs and to save the child from permanent neurological damage.

TECHNIQUES FOR SCREENING OF INBORN ERRORS OF METABOLISM

There are various techniques used for screening of inborn errors. Simple techniques, such as **chemical tests**, **paper chromatography** and **thin layer chromatography** are getting replaced with newer techniques, such as **HPLC**, **gas chromatography, tandem mass spectrometry**, etc.

BASIC CHEMICAL TESTS FOR SCREENING OF IEM

Some tests on blood and urine can be performed at the bedside or quickly in a routine laboratory. These tests are helpful in screening for many IEMs, but are not diagnostic by themselves. Detection of abnormal metabolites in urine is important for the screening of many IEMs.

The urine is an excellent source of crucial metabolites as the excess pathological metabolites in the body are excreted out in urine. Urine should be examined for the following observations before subjecting it to advanced biochemical testing. **Tables 19.1 and 19.2** outline the color and odor described in the various IEM. There are simple qualitative tests that could bring useful information about the possible metabolic error present. These tests detect specific metabolites through simple chemical reactions. **Table 19.3** describes the specialized chemical tests that can be used for the screening of IEMs. The most common tests are as follows:

- Benedict test for reducing substances
- Mucic acid test for galactose and lactose
- Ferric chloride test for PKU, histidinemia, MSUD, tyrosinemia, alkaptonuria, etc.
- 2,4-Dinitrophenylhydrazine for α-keto acids
- Cyanide nitroprusside test for cysteine and homocysteine
- Ehrlich test for porphyrins
- Toluidine blue spot test for glycosaminoglycans (GAGs)

Table 19.1: Abnormal color of urine described in IEM.

Disease	Color of the urine	Compound excreted in urine
Alkaptonuria	Dark brown or black	Homogentisic acid
Porphyrias	Red	Uroporphyrin, coproporphyrin
Hartnup disease	Blue	Indican

Table 19.2: Abnormal odor of urine described in IEM.

Disease	Odor of the urine	Compound excreted in urine
Phenylketonuria	Mouse like	Phenylacetic acid
Tyrosinemia type I	Boiled cabbage	Succinyl acetone
Maple syrup urine disease	Maple syrup, sweetish	Branched chain keto acid
Cystinuria	Sulfurous	Hydrogen sulfide
Homocystinuria	Sulfurous	Hydrogen sulfide
Isovaleric acidemia	Cheesy	Isovaleric acid

Table 19.3: Chemical test in urine and their interpretation.

Test	Color/analyte/metabolite	Disorder screened
Benedict's Test Benedict's reagent 5 mL + 8 drops of urine Boil for 2 minutes	• Green/Yellow/Orange/Brick red precipitate • Presence of reducing substances, such as fructose galactose, xylulose, homogentisic acid, 4-hydroxyphenylpyruvic acid	• Fructose: Essential fructosuria • Galactose: Galactosemia • Xylulose: Essential Pentosuria • Homogentisic acid: Alkaptonuria. • 4-hydroxyphenylpyruvic acid: Tyrosinemia I and II
Mucic acid test 25 mL of urine + 5 mL of conc. HNO_3. Heat to reduce the volume to 5 mL cool	• Crystals of mucic acid seen • Presence of galactose or lactose	Galactosemia
Ferric chloride test Add 2 drops of 10% aqueous ferric chloride to 1 mL of urine, observe the change in color	Color changes to bluish green	• Phenylketonuria, • Hyperglycinemia, • Maple syrup urine disease • Histidinemia • Alkaptonuria

Contd...

Contd...

Test	Color/analyte/metabolite	Disorder screened
Dinitrophenylhydrazine (DNPH) test Add 10 drops of DNPH reagent (100 mg DNPH +100 mL of 2N-HCl) to 1 mL of urine	• Yellow or chalky white precipitate is observed within 10 minutes • Indicates the presence of keto acids in urine	• Phenylketonuria • Maple syrup urine disease, tyrosinosis
Cyanide nitroprusside test Alkalinize 2.5 mL of urine with 2N NaOH + 1 mL of 5% sodium cyanide. After mixing, allow it to stand for 20 minutes and then add one drop of sodium nitroprusside	• A pink red to beet color within five minutes • Reaction is given by compound which possess a free sulfhydryl group or disulfide bond, therefore cystine and homocystine give this test positive	• Cystinuria • Homocystinuria
Ehrlich's aldehyde test: Equal volumes of urine and Ehrlich's aldehyde reagent are mixed	• If a pink color is formed • Raised urinary concentration of either porphobilinogen or urobilinogen in urine	Inherited porphyrias
Berry spot test/Toluidine blue-spot test/ Alcian blue spot test Urine is applied to filter paper, stained with toluidine blue, and de-stained by washing in acetic acid	• Blue color on filter paper • Presence of mucopolysaccharide	Mucopolysaccharidoses (MPS)

USE OF PAPER CHROMATOGRAPHY FOR SCREENING OF IEMS

Paper chromatography of urine sample can be used to detect a wide variety of molecules, such as amino acids, lipids, carbohydrates, hormones and many other metabolic intermediates. It is an age old technique which was predominantly used as a tool for screening of inborn errors of amino acid and carbohydrate metabolism. Principle and technique of paper chromatography is discussed in **experiment no. 14**.

The urine sample used for screening of inborn errors is run along with known standards and amino acids or sugars present in the urine are identified by their R_f values. The **Table 19.4** depicts the disorder and corresponding amino acid found in urine.

Today, newer technologies, such as HPLC, Tandem mass spectrometry are used for newborn screening as they can detect substances at very low concentrations.

Table 19.4: Urine paper chromatography for screening of IEMs.

Sl. No.	IEMs	Amino acid/sugar detected in urine
1.	Phenylketonuria	Phenylalanine
2.	Tyrosinemia	Tyrosine
3.	MSUD	Valine, leucine, isoleucine
4.	Hyperprolinemia	Proline
5.	Argininemia	arginine
6.	Glycinuria	Glycine
7.	Galactosemia	Galactose
8.	Fructosuria	fructose

VIVA QUESTIONS

1. Define inborn errors of metabolism.
2. Describe techniques for screening of IEM.
3. Describe basic chemical tests for screening of IEM.
4. Describe use of paper chromatography for screening of IEMs.
5. Name the inborn errors those can be screened by paper chromatography and give the compound excreted through urine.
6. Write advanced technique used for diagnosis/screening of inborn errors of metabolism.

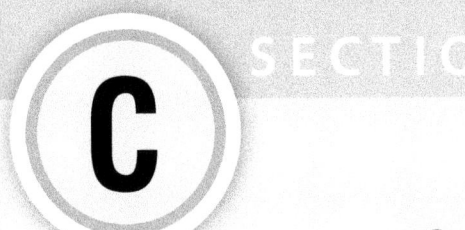

SECTION C

Quantitative Experiments Practical/DOAP

Section Outline

Experiment 20: Estimation of Blood Glucose
Experiment 21: Estimation of Blood Urea
Experiment 22: Estimation of Serum and Urine Creatinine and Creatinine Clearance
Experiment 23: Estimation of Serum Proteins, Albumin and A:G Ratio
Experiment 24: Estimation of Serum Calcium
Experiment 25: Estimation of Serum Phosphorous
Experiment 26: Estimation of Serum Bilirubin
Experiment 27: Estimation of Serum Transaminases (SGPT/ALT and SGOT/AST)
Experiment 28: Estimation of Serum Alkaline Phosphatase
Experiment 29: Estimation of Serum Total Cholesterol
Experiment 30: Estimation of Serum HDL Cholesterol
Experiment 31: Estimation of Serum Triglycerides

EXPERIMENT 20

Estimation of Blood Glucose

COMPETENCY	LEARNING OBJECTIVES
BI11.21 Demonstrate estimation of glucose, creatinine, urea and total protein in serum.	1. Describe collection of sample for blood glucose estimation 2. Describe various methods available to measure the blood glucose levels. 3. Perform estimation of blood glucose by chemical; Folin-Wu method, interpret the results and give clinical significance. 4. Perform estimation of blood glucose by enzymatic glucose oxidase peroxidase (GOD/POD) kit method, interpret the results and give clinical significance. 5. Perform estimation of capillary blood glucose test by glucometer, interpret the results and give clinical significance.

INTRODUCTION

Glucose in blood is the most frequent analyzed parameter in a clinical chemistry laboratory for screening of diabetes mellitus. Glucose concentration can be estimated in whole blood (capillary), plasma or serum. Plasma glucose is about 12 to 15% higher than whole blood glucose due to lower water content of cells (73%) of blood compared to that of plasma (94%). Plasma is preferred for estimation of glucose since whole blood is affected by proteins.

SAMPLE COLLECTION

- Blood sample is collected in **gray (ash)** colored top vacutainer tube which contains **sodium fluoride** and **potassium oxalate** mixture in the ratio of 1:3.
- When whole blood is left at room temperature after collection, glycolytic enzymes present in erythrocytes continue to utilize glucose in vitro; as a result, glycolysis reduces glucose level at the rate about 7 mg/dL/hour and low values of glucose are obtained.
- This is prevented by adding **sodium fluoride** which inhibits the enzyme enolase of glycolysis. **Potassium oxalate** acts as an anticoagulant.
- Plasma is obtained by centrifuging the blood at 2000 rpm for 10 min.

Terms Used for Blood Glucose Specimens

Depending on the time of collection, different terms are used for blood glucose specimens.
- **Fasting blood glucose**: Blood sample for glucose is withdrawn after an overnight fast (not eating at least 8 hours).

- **Post-meal or postprandial blood glucose**: Blood sample for glucose estimation is collected 2 hours after the subject has taken a normal meal.
- **Random blood glucose:** Blood sample is collected at any time of the day, without attention to the time of last food intake.

VARIOUS METHODS TO MEASURE THE BLOOD GLUCOSE LEVELS

- **Chemical methods (Folin-Wu method)** which are based on reducing property of glucose are:
  - Modified King and Asatoor method
  - Ortho-toluidine method

  As these methods, utilize the reducing property of glucose, certain other reducing substances present in blood, such as ascorbic acid and uric acid may result in higher values (up to 20–6 mg%) than the real values. Hence, this method is rarely used nowadays. Chemical methods have now been replaced by enzymatic methods.
- **Enzymatic method:** This method is more accurate and specific compared to chemical methods as the enzyme specifically act only on glucose. Either glucose oxidase, hexokinase, glucose dehydrogenase is used.

CHEMICAL (FOLIN-WU METHOD) METHOD

- **Chemical method:** Modified King and Asatoor method
- **Specimen used:** Whole Blood
- **Sample collection:** As described above

Principle

In this method, proteins in blood are precipitated with tungstic acid. The protein free filtrate-containing glucose reduces cupric ions (Cu^{2+}) to cuprous ions (Cu^+) and forms cuprous oxide (Cu_2O). Cuprous oxide then reduces phosphomolybdic acid to phosphomolybdous acid which is blue colored. The intensity of blue color is proportional to the amount of glucose present, and the color intensity is measured by using a blue filter (490 nm).

Reagents Required

- Sodium tungstate 10%
- Sulfuric acid, 2/3 N
- Alkaline copper-reagent
- Phosphomolybdic acid reagent
- Standard glucose solution: 1 mg/mL.

Procedure

- **Part 1: Preparation of protein free filtrate**—in a test tube take 7 mL of distilled water, 1 mL blood sample, 1 mL of 10% sodium tungstate solution and 1 mL of 2/3 N sulfuric acid and mix the contents let it stand for 10 minutes. Then centrifuge at 600 rpm for 10 minutes and collect the supernatant as sample. Thus, 1 mL blood is diluted to 10 mL.
- **Part 2:** Label three clean and dry Folin-Wu tubes **(Figure 20.1)** as **S (Standard) T (Test),** and **B (Blank)** and make following additions **(Table 20.1)**.

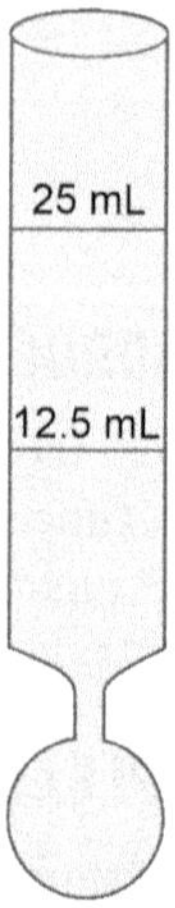

Figure 20.1: Folin-Wu tube.

Table 20.1: Estimation of blood sugar by chemical Folin Wu method:

Reagents	Blank (B)	Standard (S)	Test (T)
	2 mL distilled water	2 mL standard solution	2 mL test solution
Alkaline copper-reagent	2.0 mL	2.0 mL	2.0 mL
Keep the tubes in boiling water bath for 8 minutes and cool it. Keeping the tubes in boiling water more than 8 minutes tends to increase the reading due to excess reduction of Cu^{2+}			
Phosphomolybdic acid	2 mL	2 mL	2 mL
Add distilled water up to 25 mL mark on the Folin-Wu tube. Mix the contents by inverting tube by placing your palm tightly over the mouth of the tube and read the absorbance/optical density (OD) at 420–490 nm or blue filter against blank.			

Observations

OD B

OD S

OD T

Calculations

$$\text{Blood glucose (mg/dL)} = \frac{(OD\ T - OD\ B)}{(OD\ S - OD\ B)} \times \frac{\text{Concentration of std (mg/mL)}}{\text{Vol of sample}} \times 100\ \text{mg\%}$$

$$= \frac{OD\ T}{OD\ S} \times \frac{0.2}{0.2} \times 100\ \text{mg\%}$$

$$= \frac{OD\ T}{OD\ S} \times 100\ \text{mg\%}$$

$$= \underline{}\ \text{mg/dL}$$

ENZYMATIC METHOD

Method: GOD/POD kit Method
Specimen used: Plasma

Principle

Glucose is oxidized to gluconic acid and hydrogen peroxide in the presence of **glucose oxidase** enzyme. Hydrogen peroxide further reacts with phenol and 4-aminoantipyrine by the catalytic action of **peroxidase** to form a red-colored quinoneimine dye complex. The intensity of the color is directly proportional to the concentration of glucose present in blood. The absorbance of color is measured colorimetrically at 56 nm and compared with that of a standard treated similarly.

Reagents

- **Glucose reagent:** Glucose oxidase, peroxidase, 4-amino antipyrine and phenol
- **Glucose standard solution:** Concentration = 1 mg/mL

Procedure

Take clean and dry test tubes and label them as Blank (B), Standard (S) and Test (T) and make following additions (**Table 20.2**).

Table 20.2: Estimation of blood glucose by enzymatic glucose oxidase peroxidase (GOD/POD) method.

Reagents	Blank (B)	Standard (S)	Test (T)
Glucose reagent	1.0 mL	1.0 mL	1.0 mL
Distilled water	10 µL	-	-
Glucose standard	-	10 µL	-
Plasma sample	-	-	10 µL

Mix well and incubate at 37°C for 10 minutes. Read colorimetrically at 530 nm/green filter.

Observations

OD B

OD S

OD T

Calculations

Plasma glucose (mg/dL) = $\dfrac{OD\ T}{OD\ S} \times 100$ mg

= _____ mg/dL

Certain laboratories express glucose concentration in SI units (Millimoles/liter). The values in mmol/L can be derived through the following formula:

Plasma glucose *(mmol/L)* = $\dfrac{(\text{Concentration in mg /dL})}{(\text{molecular weight})} \times 10$

= _____ mmol/L

(Molecular weight is 180)

Normal Reference Range

Fasting plasma glucose: 70–110 mg/dL
Postprandial plasma glucose: Less than 140 mg/dL
Random plasma glucose: 70–140 mg/dL

Result

Plasma glucose = _____ mg/dL

Clinical Significance

When blood glucose concentration is higher than the normal range, it is known as **hyperglycemia** and the value is lower than the normal limit, it is called as **hypoglycemia**.

a. Hyperglycemia is found in following conditions:
   1. Diabetes mellitus
   2. Hyperfunction of the pituitary and adrenal gland
   3. Diseases of pancreas, such as pancreatitis and carcinoma
   4. Meningitis, encephalitis, shock
   5. Emotional states, such as fear, anger and anxiety
b. Hypoglycemia is found in following conditions:
   1. Insulin over dose in diabetic patients
   2. Tumors of pancreas (insulinoma) affecting beta cells
   3. Glycogen storage diseases
   4. Hypoactivity of thyroid, adrenals and pituitary glands

CAPILLARY BLOOD GLUCOSE TEST BY GLUCOMETER

Nowadays, a small portable device, i.e., "Glucometer"**(Figure 20.2)** is used to blood glucose monitoring outside the clinical laboratory. It measures capillary blood glucose levels within seconds. This instrument is based on the principles of **enzymatic assessment** of blood glucose. Glucometer is commonly being used not only by physician at his clinic and hospitals as a bedside measure of blood glucose monitoring; it is common household item which is extensively used by patient himself to estimate blood glucose. Glucometer is an example of point of care testing (POCT). The kit of glucometer contains following items in it:

❖ Instrument glucometer
❖ Test strip
❖ Needle (Lancet)
❖ Alcohol swab

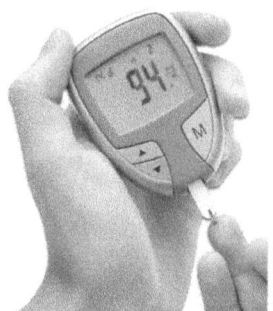

Figure 20.2: Glucometer.

Working Principle of Glucometer

- A little drop of whole blood that is to be tested is put on a glucometer test strip.
- Glucometer test strip contains an enzyme (glucose oxidase-peroxidase) in dry form at one of its ends. This enzyme then reacts with the glucose in the blood sample and creates an acid called gluconic acid.
- The gluconic acid thus formed then reacts with another chemical in the testing strip called ferricyanide. The ferricyanide and the gluconic acid then combine with each other and forms ferrocyanide.
- Immediately as the ferrocyanide has been formed, the device glucometer runs an electronic current through the blood sample on the strip.
- The current thus produced is capable of reading the ferrocyanide and identifying the amount of glucose present in the blood sample on the testing strip. This number is the only value that is displayed on the screen of the glucometer.
- Whole blood glucose concentration is 10 to 15% lower than the plasma or serum glucose concentration.

Steps to Perform Glucose Estimation Using Glucometer

- Turn on the glucometer.
- Place a test strip in the socket correctly
- Place the lancet in lancet holder
- Prick the finger using lancing device
- Squeeze your finger until it has produced a sufficient-size drop
- Place the drop of blood on the strip
- Blot your finger with the alcohol swab to stop the bleeding
- Wait a few moments for the glucometer to generate a reading

Advantages of Glucometer

- It is quick and the result is available as the earliest, anywhere and anytime.
- This becomes important in situations, such as emergency departments, operation theaters, intensive care units, etc., where time is a critical factor.

ASSESSMENT QUESTION

Q. Case-based quantitative estimation.
A 50-year-old lady attended outpatient clinic with history of passing large volumes of urine at frequent intervals, unusual thirst and overeating and a feeling of weight loss for the past 3 months. Identify the case and do the estimation of relevant parameter. Express your result and interpret.

VIVA QUESTIONS

1. What are the methods used to estimate glucose in the blood? Which is the best method among them? Why?
2. How will you collect blood sample for glucose estimation?
3. Give the principle of glucose oxidase method of blood glucose estimation.
4. What are the normal blood glucose values?
5. What are the causes of hyperglycemia?
6. What are the causes of hypoglycemia?
7. What is the use of glucometer?
8. What is the principle of glucometer?
9. Which are the advantages of glucometer as point of care testing?

EXPERIMENT 21

Estimation of Blood Urea

COMPETENCY	LEARNING OBJECTIVES
BI11.21 Demonstrate estimation of glucose, creatinine, urea and total protein in serum.	1. Perform estimation of blood urea, interpret the results and give clinical significance. 2. Describe enzymatic Berthelot reaction (Kit method).

INTRODUCTION

Urea is the end product of protein catabolism. Deamination of amino acids release ammonia which is detoxified in the liver to form urea. More than 90% of urea produced is excreted through kidney in urine and the rest through GI tract and skin. Urea is freely filtered through glomeruli, hence dysfunction of glomeruli whereby filtration is affected, urea tends to accumulate in plasma and estimation of plasma urea gives idea regarding renal function.

Plasma urea concentration depends upon dietary protein intake, hepatic function and kidney function. Urea estimation is one of the most widely applied tests for kidney function evaluation. The test is frequently tested in conjunction with creatinine determination for diagnosis renal uremia (abnormally high levels of waste products in the blood due to impaired renal function). In some laboratories, blood urea is represented as **'blood urea nitrogen' (BUN)**.

Urea concentration can be estimated in whole blood, plasma or serum depending on the method. The concentration of urea in whole blood is slightly less than that of plasma or serum.

ESTIMATION OF BLOOD UREA

Chemical method: Diacetyl monoxime (DAM) method
Specimen used: Blood
Sample Collection: Collect whole blood in a yellow color-coded vacuum evacuated tube. It prevents the blood from clotting.

Principle

Under acidic condition and in presence of ferric ions and thiosemicarbazide, urea reacts with diacetyl monoxime, to form a pink-colored complex which is measured colorimetrically at 530 nm green filter. The intensity of the color is directly proportional to the concentration of urea present in blood. A standard urea solution is treated similarly and color intensities are compared.

Reagents

- Sodium tungstate, 10%
- Sulfuric acid, 2/3 N
- Urea color reagent: Diacetyl monoxime, thiosemicarbazide and ferric chloride.
- Standard urea solution (0.03 mg/mL)

Procedure

- **Part 1: Preparation of protein-free filtrate**—in a test tube take 3.4 mL of distilled water, 0.1 mL blood sample, 1.5 mL of 10% TCA. Mix the contents let it stand for 10 minutes. Then centrifuge at 600 rpm for 10 min and collect the supernatant as sample. Thus, 1 mL blood is diluted to 50 mL.
- **Part 2:** Label three clean and dry test tubes as **S (Standard)**, **T (Test)**, and **B (Blank)** and proceed as given in the **Table 21.1**

Table 21.1: Procedure for blood urea estimation.

Reagents	Blank (B)	Standard (S)	Test (T)
	1 mL Distilled water	1 mL Urea standard solution	1 mL Protein free filtrate
Urea color reagent	5.0 mL	5.0 mL	5.0 mL

Keep these three tubes in boiling water bath for 20 minutes. Cool to room temperature. Read colorimetrically at 530 nm/green filter.

Observations

OD S

OD T

OD B

Calculations

Serum urea (mg/dL) $= \dfrac{(OD\ T - OD\ B)}{(OD\ S - OD\ .B)} \times \dfrac{\text{Conc. of std}}{\text{Vol. of sample}} \times 100$

$= \dfrac{OD\ T}{OD\ S} \times \dfrac{0.03}{0.02} \times 100$

$= \dfrac{OD\ T}{OD\ S} \times 150$

$=$ _____ mg/dL

Blood urea nitrogen (mg/dL) $= \dfrac{\text{Blood urea}}{2.14}$

$=$ _____ mg/dL

Results

Blood urea = _____ mg/dL
Blood urea nitrogen = _____ mg/dL

Normal Reference Range

- Blood urea: 15–40 mg/dL
- Blood urea nitrogen: 10–20 mg/dL

Clinical Significance

Elevated levels of urea (Azotemia) are observed in prerenal, renal, and postrenal conditions. The term 'uremia' is used to refer to elevated blood urea levels due to renal pathology.

- **Prerenal condition:** Diabetes mellitus, dehydration, cardiac failure, severe burns (due to excess protein breakdown), high fever, etc.
  - Decrease in blood volume occurs in dehydration due to prolonged diarrhea, vomiting, burns, etc.
  - The decrease blood volume leads to low blood pressure, which decreases effective filtration rate in glomeruli and reduces filtration of urea.
  - Increased tissue protein breakdown occurs in diabetes and in different types of fevers.
- **Renal condition:** Disease of kidneys for example in nephritis, acute glomerulonephritis and renal tuberculosis.
- **Post-renal condition:** Enlargement of prostate, stones in urinary tract, stricture of the urethra, tumor of the bladder
- The clinical significance of the urea level in plasma is usually determined in conjugation with the plasma creatinine level. In prerenal azotemia, an increase in the plasma urea level is usually associated with a normal plasma creatinine level, whereas in postrenal azotemia, there is an increase in both the urea and the plasma creatinine levels.
- Decreased values have been reported in severe liver disease, and protein malnutrition and pregnancy.

ENZYMATIC KIT METHOD: BERTHELOT REACTION

- In this method to estimate blood urea, blood plasma or serum is used.
- It is based on the principle that urea is hydrolyzed into ammonia and carbon dioxide by enzyme urease.
- The ammonia produced is measured photometrically after its reaction with phenol in the presence of hypochlorite (Berthelot reaction).
- This blue color reaction product is determined photometrically. Intensity of the color formed is directly proportional to the amount of urea present in the sample.
- This method is widely used because of the absolute specificity of enzyme urease.

Released ammonia can also be quantified by various other methods.

ASSESSMENT QUESTION

Q. Case-based quantitative estimation.
A 4-year-old lady presented in the clinic complaining of nausea, weakness, and swelling on feet and ankles. She had a history of recurrent urinary tract infection in the last 2 weeks, for which she was treated with antibiotics. She felt that her urine output has also decreased over the last one week. She is a diabetic for the last 4 years for which she is taking medicines. Her recent investigation showed increased serum creatinine level. The serum sample of the patient is provided to you. Identify the case and do the estimation of other relevant parameter. Express your result and interpret.

VIVA QUESTIONS

1. What is the method used to estimate urea in the blood? Give its principle.
2. What are the other methods of urea estimation?
3. Give the normal values of blood urea.
4. What is the most common indication of doing blood urea estimation?
5. Can blood urea level decrease?
6. What is uremia? What are the different causes of uremia?
7. What are the prerenal causes of uremia? Explain the mechanism of the causation uremia in these conditions.
8. Mention three renal causes of uremia.
9. Mention three post-renal causes of uremia. Explain the mechanism.

EXPERIMENT 22

Estimation of Serum and Urine Creatinine and Creatinine Clearance

COMPETENCY		LEARNING OBJECTIVES
BI11.7	Demonstrate the estimation of serum creatinine and creatinine clearance.	1. Perform estimation of serum creatinine, interpret the results and give clinical significance.
BI11.22	Calculate albumin: Globulin (A/G) ratio and creatinine clearance.	2. Perform estimation of urine creatinine, interpret the results and give clinical significance.
		3. Determine creatinine clearance and give its clinical significance.

INTRODUCTION

Creatine is synthesized in liver and kidney from amino acids; glycine, arginine and methionine. It is carried by blood to skeletal muscle and brain and converted to creatine phosphate. Creatine phosphate serves as the storage form of energy in muscle. Energy needed for muscle contraction is provided by ATP break down to form ADP. ATP is regenerated from ADP by hydrolysis of creatine phosphate by creatine kinase to creatine which in turn converted by spontaneous dehydration into creatinine. The amount of creatinine produced is related to the muscle mass and remains constant in an individual unless muscle mass changes.

Creatinine excreted by kidney where it is freely filtered through the glomerulus with negligible tubular reabsorption and secreted in the tubules to a minor degree. Serum creatinine level is a sensitive index of renal function and creatinine clearance is a good measure of GFR.

ESTIMATION OF SERUM CREATININE

Method: Chemical method; Jaffe's method
Specimen: Serum
Serum sample collection: Collect blood in a red-colored top vacutainer tube. Then allow the blood to clot the blood by leaving it undisturbed at room temperature for 15–6 minutes. Remove the clot by centrifuging at 1,000–2,000 RPM for 10 minutes. The resulting supernatant is serum.

Principle

Picric acid in an alkaline medium reacts with creatinine to form an orange-colored complex of creatinine picrate. The intensity of which measured colorimetrically at 530 nm. Intensity of the color formed is directly proportional to the amount of creatinine present in the sample.

Reagents

- Sodium tungstate 10%
- Sulfuric acid, 2/3 N
- Picric acid solution, 0.04 M/L (0.916 g of hydrated picric acid/100 mL distilled water)
- NaOH, 0.75N (3 g/100 mL water)
- Standard creatinine solution (0.01 mg/mL in 0.1 N HCl).

Procedure

- **Part 1: Preparation of protein free filtrate (PFF):** In a test tube, take 1 mL of distilled water + 1 mL serum (or plasma) + 1 mL of 5% sodium tungstate +1 mL of 2/3 N sulfuric acid and mix the contents let it stand for 10 minutes and centrifuge at 600 rpm for 10 min and collect the supernatant as sample. Thus 4 mL protein free filtrate contains 1 mL of serum sample.
- **Part 2:** Label three clean and dry test tubes as **S (Standard) T (Test),** and **B (Blank)** and proceed as given in the **Table 22.1.**

Table 22.1: Procedure for serum creatinine estimation.

Reagents	Blank (B)	Standard (S)	Test (T)
	3 mL distilled water	3 mL creatinine standard solution	3 mL PFF
Picric acid (0.04 M)	1 mL	1 mL	1 mL
NaOH (0.75N)	1 mL	1 mL	1 mL

Mix well and keep at room temperature for 15 minutes. Read OD colorimetrically at 530 nm/ green filter.

Observations

$$OD\ S$$
$$OD\ T$$
$$OD\ B$$

Calculations

Serum creatinine (mg/dL)
$$= \frac{(OD\ T - OD\ B)}{(OD\ S - OD\ B)} \times \frac{Conc.\ of\ std.}{Vol.\ of\ sample} \times 100$$

$$= \frac{OD\ T}{OD\ S} \times \frac{0.03}{0.75} \times 100$$

$$= \frac{OD\ T}{OD\ S} \times 4$$

$$= \underline{\qquad}\ mg/dL$$

Results: Serum creatinine = _____ mg/dL

Normal Reference Range

- Males: 0.7–1.5 mg/dL
- Females: 0.5–1.1 mg/dL

Other Method

Enzymatic method (using creatinase, peroxidase)

ESTIMATION OF URINE CREATININE

Method: Chemical method; Jaffe's method
Specimen: Urine
Urine sample collection: A 24-hour urine sample is collected for estimating urinary creatinine. The bladder must be emptied before starting the collection of 24-hour urine and this urine is discarded. Time is noted. Thereafter all urine must be collected in a special container using chloroform as preservative until the end of 24 hours. Dilute the urine 10 times (1 mL urine + 9 mL distilled water) prior to estimation due to high concentration of creatinine in urine.

Principle

As discussed for serum creatinine estimation

Reagent

As discussed for serum creatinine estimation

Procedure

- Dilute 1 mL urine to 10 ml with distilled water.
- Label three clean and dry test tubes as **S (Standard) T (Test)**, and **B (Blank)** and proceed as given in the **Table 22.2**.

Table 22.2: Procedure for urine creatinine estimation.

Reagents	Blank (B)	Standard (S)	Test (T)
	5 mL Distilled water	5 mL Creatinine standard solution	5 mL Diluted urine
Picric acid (0.04 M)	2 mL	2 mL	2 mL
NaOH (0.75 N)	2 mL	2 mL	2 mL

Mix well and keep at room temperature for 15 minutes. Read OD colorimetrically at 530 nm/green filter.

Observations

OD S

OD T

OD B

Calculations

Serum creatinine (mg/dL)
$$= \frac{(OD\ T - OD\ B)}{(OD\ S - OD\ .B)} \times \frac{\text{Conc. of std.}}{\text{Vol. of sample}} \times 100$$

$$= \frac{OD\ T}{OD\ S} \times \frac{0.05}{0.5} \times 100$$

$$= \frac{OD\ T}{OD\ S} \times 10$$

Results = _____ mg/dL

Normal Reference Range

- Males: 1–3.0 g/L
- Females: 1.0–2 g/L

DETERMINATION OF CREATININE CLEARANCE

Creatinine clearance test is widely used as a measure of the GFR and it is decreased in advanced renal failure. Creatinine clearance is defined as the volume of plasma cleared off creatinine in 1 minute. The creatinine level in blood and urine are measured for the estimation of creatinine clearance. The serum collection must be within 24 hours of urine collection.

Procedure

At a defined point of time, the patient is asked to void urine and this sample is discarded. The rest of the urine subsequently voided over a prescribed time period of 24 hours is then collected. A blood sample is collected in between. Creatinine is estimated in both the samples and then its clearance is calculated using following formula:

Creatinine clearance (mL/minute) $\frac{UV}{P}$

Where:
U = Urine creatinine (mg/dL)
V = Urine flow in mL/minute
P = Plasma/serum creatinine (mg/dL)

Creatinine clearance can also be calculated by using **Cockcroft-Gault formula**, if serum creatinine concentration, age, and weight of an individual are known. K = 0.85 for women and 1 for men

Estimated creatinine clearance mL/min = $\frac{(140-age) \times weight (kg) \times K}{72 \times serum\ creatinine\ (mg/dL)}$

Results

Creatinine clearance = _____ mL/minute

Normal Reference Range

Gender	Serum	Urine (24 hours collection)	Creatinine clearance
Males	0.7–1.5 mg/dL	1–3.0 g/L	95–140 mL/min
Females	0.5–1.1 mg/dL	1–2 g/L	80–115 mL/min

(Laboratory methods and instrumentation can affect the normal value given)

CLINICAL SIGNIFICANCE

- The creatinine levels are taken as more reliable indicators of kidney function than blood urea or uric acid. This is because, unlike other substances, the creatinine level is unaffected by diet, exercise or hormonal factors.
- Increased serum levels are seen in renal dysfunction reduced renal blood flow (shock, dehydration, congestive heart failure) diabetes mellitus and other renal diseases.
- Measurement of creatinine is not; however, a sensitive index for the diagnosis of early renal failure since it may remain within normal limits at a glomerular filtration rate reduced to half normal value.
- Renal function can be evaluated by measuring the glomerular filtration rate (GFR). Creatinine clearance values are close to glomerular filtration rate (GFR). Creatinine clearance provides a more accurate assessment and can be calculated from serum creatinine and creatinine in 24 hours urine collected.
- Creatinine clearance values are decreased in impaired renal function and so provide a rough measure of glomerular damage. Creatinine clearance is often used for the initial evaluation of renal diseases, such as glomerulonephritis.
- It can also be used to monitor the progression of chronic renal failure, the response to therapy or help to decide when to dialysis in patients with decline renal function.
- Low serum creatinine is not significant. It is associated with muscle wasting diseases (muscular dystrophy).

ASSESSMENT QUESTION

Q. Case-based quantitative estimation.

A 50-year-old man, known case of hypertension and renal failure admitted in hospital with complains of nausea and vomiting. He had high-grade fever and fewer intakes from last week. On investigations, his blood urea was 70 mg/dL and urine output 800 mL/day. What other test you will perform to diagnose the disease in this patient. Choose and estimate appropriate biochemical parameter. Express your result and interpret.

VIVA QUESTIONS

1. What is creatine and what is the importance of estimating serum creatinine level?
2. What is the method used to estimate creatinine in the blood? Give its principle.
3. What is the normal serum creatinine level?
4. What is the reason for low creatinine concentrations in females than in males?
5. Why creatinine is preferred than blood urea in assessing renal function?
6. What is the importance of increased serum creatinine level?
7. Define clearance. What is normal creatinine clearance?

EXPERIMENT 23

Estimation of Serum Proteins, Albumin and A:G Ratio

COMPETENCY	LEARNING OBJECTIVES
BI11.8 Demonstrate estimation of serum proteins, albumin and A:G ratio. **BI11.21** Demonstrate estimation of glucose, creatinine, urea and total protein in serum. **BI11.22** Calculate albumin: Globulin ratio and creatinine clearance.	1. Perform estimation of serum total proteins 2. Perform estimation of serum albumin 3. Calculate A:G ratio. 4. Interpret the results and give clinical significance of serum proteins, albumin and A:G ratio

INTRODUCTION

Proteins are the most abundant biomolecule in the cell. Blood contains many proteins. Albumin, globulin and fibrinogen are the major proteins present in the blood or plasma. Serum proteins consist of albumin and globulin, fibrinogen is absent because fibrinogen is consumed during clotting process. Albumin consists of approximately 60% of the total plasma proteins in the body, the other major part being globulin. Estimation of total proteins and A:G ratio is routinely done to assess the liver and renal functions.

ESTIMATION OF SERUM TOTAL PROTEINS

Method: Biuret method. It is the most commonly used method for estimation of total protein in clinical lab. This method is called biuret method because a compound known as biuret reacts with cupric ion to give similar color.
Specimen: Serum
Serum sample collection: Collect blood in a red-colored top vacutainer tube. Then allow the blood to clot the blood by leaving it undisturbed at room temperature for 15–6 minutes. Remove the clot by centrifuging at 1,000–2,000 RPM for 10 minutes. The resulting supernatant is serum.

Principle

When serum is treated with biuret reagent, the peptide bonds of proteins react with cupric ions in alkaline medium of biuret reagent to form a violet-colored complex. The optical density is measured colorimetrically at 530 nm. A standard protein solution is also treated similarly and the color intensities are compared.

Reagents

- **Biuret reagent:** Sodium potassium tartrate + copper sulphate, potassium iodide and sodium hydroxide.
- Sodium chloride 0.9 % (Normal saline)
- **Protein standard solution:** Concentration = 5 mg/mL

Procedure

- **Dilution of serum:** Take 0.2 mL of serum sample. Add 3.8 mL normal saline and mix.
- Label three clean and dry test tubes as **S (Standard) T (Test),** and **B (Blank)** and proceed as given in the **Table 23.1**

Table 23.1 : Procedure for serum protein estimation.

Reagents	Blank (B)	Standard (S)	Test (T)
	1 mL Normal saline	1 mL Protein standard	1mL Diluted serum
Biuret reagent	5.0 mL	5.0 mL	5.0 mL

Mix and keep at RT for 10 minutes and read colorimetrically at 530 nm/green filter.

Observations

OD S

OD T

OD B

Calculations

Serum total proteins (g/dL)
$$= \frac{(OD\ T - OD\ B)}{(OD\ S - OD\ .B)} \times \frac{Conc.\ of\ std.}{Vol.\ of\ serum} \times 100 \times \frac{1}{1000}$$

$$= \frac{OD\ T}{OD\ S} \times \frac{5}{0.05} \times 100 \times \frac{1}{1000}$$

$$= \frac{OD\ T}{OD\ S} \times 10$$

$$= \underline{\hspace{2cm}} g/dL$$

Other Methods Used for Estimation of Total Serum Protein

- Lowry method
- Kjeldahl method
- Turbidimetric method
- Nephelometric method

ESTIMATION OF SERUM ALBUMIN

Method: Bromocresol green (BCG) method
Sample used: Serum
Serum sample collection: As discussed for total serum protein estimation

Principle

Albumin binds with the bromocresol green (BCG) in buffer medium to form a green-colored complex. The color intensity measured colorimetrically at 620 nm. The intensity of color formed is directly proportional to the amount of albumin present in the sample. BCG is the dye of choice because it is bound tightly to albumin and it is not displaced by bilirubin.

Reagents

- Bromocresol green dye
- Normal saline
- Albumin standard solution: Concentration = 5 mg/mL

Procedure

- **Dilution of serum:** Take 0.2 mL of serum sample. Add 1.8 mL normal saline and mix.
- Label three clean and dry test tubes as **S (Standard) T (Test)**, and **B (Blank)** and proceed as given in the **Table 23.2.**

Table 23.2: Procedure for serum albumin estimation.

Reagents	Blank (B)	Standard (S)	Test (T)
	0.2 mL Normal saline	0.2 mL Albumin standard	0.2 mL Diluted serum
Working BCG dye	5.0 mL	5.0 mL	5.0 mL

Mix and keep at RT for 10 minutes and read colorimetrically at 620 nm/red filter.

Observations

OD S

OD T

OD B

Calculations

Serum albumin (g/dL)

$$= \frac{(OD\ T - OD\ B)}{(OD\ S - OD\ B)} \times \frac{Conc.\ of\ std.}{Vol.\ of\ sample} \times 100 \times \frac{1}{1000}$$

$$= \frac{OD\ T}{OD\ S} \times \frac{1}{0.02} \times 100 \times \frac{1}{1000}$$

$$= \frac{OD\ T}{OD\ S} \times 5$$

= _____ g/dL

Serum globulin (g/dL) = Total proteins (g/dL) - Albumin (g/dL)

= _____ g/dL

A/G ratio = $\frac{Albumin\ (g/dL)}{Globulin\ (g/dL)}$ = _____

Result

Serum total protein	= _____	g/dL
Serum albumin	= _____	g/dL
Serum globulin	= _____	g/dL
A/G ratio	= _____	

Normal Reference Range

Total proteins: 6.0–8.0 g/dL
Serum albumin :   3.7–5.3 g/dL
Serum globulin :   2.3–3.6 g/dL
A/G ratio: 1.0–2.3

CLINICAL SIGNIFICANCE

Hyperproteinemia: Increase in total serum proteins is either due to increase production of globulins or due to relative decrease in plasma water concentration (hemoconcentration).
- Rise in globulins is associated with conditions like multiple myeloma and chronic infections like tuberculosis.
- Hemoconcentration is seen in conditions like dehydration due to inadequate water intake or excessive water loss as in severe vomiting, diarrhea or fever.

Hypoproteinemia: Decrease in total serum proteins is often due to decreased serum albumin concentration associated with following conditions:
- Decreased intake—protein-energy malnutrition
- Decreased synthesis—chronic liver diseases
- Decreased dietary absorption—malabsorption syndrome
- Increased loss—nephrotic syndrome, chronic glomerulonephritis, diabetic nephropathy and increased fluid loss through skin during extensive burns.
- Hypoproteinemia may also be associated with hemodilution due to water intoxication or salt retention.

Significance of A/G ratio

The A/G ratio is reversed either due to increase in globulins or decrease in albumin. It is reversed in conditions, such as multiple myeloma, chronic liver diseases and renal disorders.
- In multiple myeloma γ-globulin fraction is increased thus reversing the A/G ratio.
- In renal disorders, there is a loss of albumin whereas globulins are retained, thus reversing A/G ratio.
- In chronic liver diseases, albumin fraction is decreased resulting in reversal of A/G ratio.

ASSESSMENT QUESTION

Q. Case-based quantitative estimation.
A 6-year-old boy was brought to pediatrics OPD by mother with complaints of puffiness of face, generalized swelling of body with decreased urine output. The serum sample of the patient is provided to you. Estimation of creatinine and urea has been done already. Identify the case and do the estimation of other relevant parameters. Express your result and interpret.

VIVA QUESTIONS

1. Name the method used in the estimation of total protein.
2. What are the normal levels of total proteins, albumin, globulins and A:G ratio?
3. How will you collect serum sample?
4. Mention the common causes of hyperproteinemia.
5. What is the importance of A:G ratio?

EXPERIMENT 24

Estimation of Serum Calcium

COMPETENCY	LEARNING OBJECTIVES
BI11.11 Demonstrate the estimation of calcium.	1. Perform estimation of the serum calcium, interpret the results and give its clinical significance.

INTRODUCTION

Calcium is the most abundant mineral in the body. The adult human body contains about 1 to 1.4 kg of calcium. About 99% the body's calcium is present in bone and teeth together with phosphate as the hydroxyapatite crystals. Only small amount of total body calcium is in the plasma. In serum, calcium exists equally in a free ionized form and in a bound form with albumin.

Intracellular calcium participates in muscle contraction, hormone secretion, and second messenger of hormone action, metabolic activities and enzyme actions.

ESTIMATION OF SERUM CALCIUM

Method: O-cresolphthalein complexone (OCPC) method (colorimetric method)
Specimen: Serum
Serum sample collection: Collect blood in a red-colored top vacutainer tube. Then allow the blood to clot the blood by leaving it undisturbed at room temperature for 15–6 minutes. Remove the clot by centrifuging at 1,000–2,000 RPM for 10 minutes. The resulting supernatant is serum.

Principle

In alkaline medium, calcium binds with o-cresolphthalein complexone (O-CPC) to produce a purple-colored complex. Intensity of color complex is directly proportional to the concentration of calcium present in the sample, which is measured colorimetrically at 530 nm filter.

Reagents

- **Calcium standard solution (10 mg/dL):** 250 mg of anhydrous calcium carbonate +50 mL HCl +250 mL DDW.
- **Working calcium standard:** 10 mL stock + 100 mL DDW.

- **Buffer:** Dissolve 210 g of diethanolamine and 60 g of urea in about 900 mL of double distilled water (DDW). Adjust to pH 11.7 with acetic acid and dilute to 100 mL with DDW. It is stable for 2 months.
- **Color (OCPC) reagent:** Dissolve 64 mg of O-cresolphthalein complexone + 1.16 g of 8-hydroxyquinoline + 2.5 mL of acetic acid in 250 mL of 2.5% ethanol.
- **Working color reagent:** Two volumes of buffer and 1 volume of color reagent. Use only on the day of preparation.

Procedure

Label three clean and dry test tubes as **S (Standard) T (Test),** and **B (Blank)** and proceed as given in the **Table 24.1.**

Table 24.1: Procedure for serum calcium estimation.

Reagents	Blank (B)	Standard (S)	Test (T)
	0.05 mL Distilled water	0.05 mL Calcium standard	0.05 mL Serum
Color reagent	5 mL	5 mL	5 mL

Mix well and keep at RT for 5 minutes. Read colorimetrically at 530 nm/green filter.

Observations

OD S

OD T

OD B

Calculations

Serum calcium (mg/dL)

$$= \frac{(OD\ T - OD\ B)}{(OD\ S - OD\ B)} \times \frac{Conc.\ of\ std.}{Vol.\ of\ sample} \times 100$$

$$= \frac{OD\ T}{OD\ S} \times \frac{0.005}{0.05} \times 100$$

$$= \frac{OD\ T}{OD\ S} \times 10$$

Result: Serum calcium = _____ mg/dL

Normal reference range: 9–11 mg/dL

Other Methods for Estimation of Serum Calcium

- Arsenazo III dye method
- Clark and Collip method: Titration method

Clinical Significance

Serum calcium concentration is affected by
- Defective absorption of calcium from gastrointestinal tract
- Altered parathyroid hormone secretion
- Changes in serum phosphorous concentration
- Changes in serum protein concentration
- Altered pH

- ❖ **Hypercalcemia:** Hypercalcemia occurs due to excessive release of calcium from skeleton, intestine or kidney into extracellular fluid. Chronic hypercalcemia causes renal tubular damage and increases the risk of renal stone formation. Different conditions leading to hypercalcemia are:
  - Hyperparathyroidism
  - Hypervitaminosis D
  - Neoplastic disease of bone
  - Osteolytic disease like multiple myeloma.
- ❖ **Hypocalcemia:** Low levels of serum calcium below 7 mg% causes tetany resulting in serve convulsions and cardiac arrhythmias, progressing to seizures and death. Chronic hypocalcemia may cause psychiatric symptoms, bone pain and fragility, dental abnormalities, and cataract formation. Hypocalcemia is found in:
  - Hypoparathyroidism
  - Hypovitaminosis D (rickets, osteomalacia)
  - Advanced renal failure
  - Malabsorption

ASSESSMENT QUESTION

Q. Case-based quantitative estimation.

A 65 year old lady was complaining of weakness, numbness, and tingling sensation in lower limbs, tremors and muscle cramps. Estimation of serum inorganic phosphorous has been already done. The serum sample of the patient is provided to you. Identify the case and do the estimation of other relevant parameter. Express your result and interpret.

VIVA QUESTIONS

1. Mention two methods for estimating calcium in the serum.
2. What are the different functions offered by calcium in the body?
3. What is the normal total serum calcium level?
4. Mention the common causes of hypercalcemia.
5. What are the causes of hypocalcemia?

EXPERIMENT 25

Estimation of Serum Phosphorous

COMPETENCY	LEARNING OBJECTIVES
BI11.11 Demonstrate the estimation of phosphorous.	1. Perform estimation of the serum inorganic phosphorous, interpret the results and give its clinical significance.

INTRODUCTION

Phosphorus mainly combines with calcium and is essential for bone formation. It plays a role in various metabolic pathways, regulating acid-base balance. It is an integral component of the energy currency of the cell, ATP.

ESTIMATION OF SERUM INORGANIC PHOSPHOROUS

Method: Colorimetric method: Fiske-Subbarow method
Specimen: Serum
Serum sample collection: Collect blood in a red-colored top vacutainer tube. Then allow the blood to clot the blood by leaving it undisturbed at room temperature for 15–6 minutes. Remove the clot by centrifuging at 1,000–2,000 RPM for 10 minutes. The resulting supernatant is serum.

Principle

The protein free filtrate of serum is obtained by treating serum with TCA. The inorganic phosphorous present in protein free filtrate reacts with molybdic acid to form hexavalent phosphomolybdic acid. The hexavalent molybdenum of the phosphomolybdic acid is then reduced by amino-naphthol-sulfonic acid (ANSA) to give a blue-colored complex. The absorbance of which is measured colorimetrically at 660 nm/red filter. A standard phosphorous solution is treated similarly and the color intensities are compared.

Reagents

- About 10% Trichloroacetic acid (TCA)
- Molybdic acid reagent (2.5% ammonium molybdate in 3N sulfuric acid (H_2SO_4)
- Amino-naphthol-sulfonic acid (ANSA) reagent
- Phosphate standard solution (0.008 mg/mL)

Procedure

- **Preparation of protein free filtrate:** In a test tube, take 9 mL of 10% TCA and add 1 mL of serum drop wise. Mix and allow the contents to stand for 5 minutes and filter to obtain a protein free filtrate (PFF).
- **Color development:** Label three clean and dry test tubes as **S (Standard) T (Test),** and **B (Blank)** and proceed as given in the **Table 25.1**.

Table 25.1: Procedure for serum phosphorous estimation.

Reagents	Blank (B)	Standard (S)	Test (T)
	2.5 mL Distilled water	2.5 mL Phosphorus standard	2.5 mL Protein free filtrate
Molybdic acid reagent	0.5 mL	0.5 mL	0.5 mL
ANSA	0.2 mL	0.2 mL	0.2 mL
Distilled water	1.8 mL	1.8 mL	1.8 mL

Mix well and keep at RT for 5 minutes. Read colorimetrically at 660 nm/red filter.

Observations

OD S

OD T

OD B

Calculations

Serum phosphorous (mg/dL) $= \dfrac{(OD\ T - OD\ B)}{(OD\ S - OD\ .B)} \times \dfrac{Conc.\ of\ std.}{Vol.\ of\ sample} \times 100$

$= \dfrac{OD\ T}{OD\ S} \times \dfrac{0.02}{0.25} \times 100$

$= \dfrac{OD\ T}{OD\ S} \times 8$

= _____ mg/dL

Result: Serum phosphorous = _____ mg/dL

Reference Range

Adults: 2.5–4.5 mg/dL
Children: 4–6 mg/dL

Other Methods for Estimation of Serum Phosphorous

Several enzymatic methods have been described for measuring serum phosphorus.

Clinical Significance

- **Hyperphosphatemia:** Elevated phosphate causes a decrease in serum calcium concentration which may lead to tetany and seizures. An increase in serum phosphorus is seen in:
  - **Renal failure:** A decrease in GFR hinder excretion of phosphate in urine leading to hyperphosphatemia
  - **Hypoparathyroidism and acromegaly:** Enhances tubular reabsorption of phosphates

- Hypervitaminosis D
- ❖ **Hypophosphatemia:** Clinical manifestations of hypophosphatemia depend on duration and extent of the deficiency. Since phosphate is a component of ATP, cellular functions are impaired in hypophosphatemia. It leads to muscle weakness, respiratory failure, decreased cardiac output. At very low concentration (below 0.5 mg %) rhabdomyolysis, lysis of RBC, mental confusion and even coma may occur. Chronic hypophosphatemia causes rickets in children and osteomalacia in adults. Hypophosphatemia is seen in:
  - Hyperparathyroidism
  - Hypovitaminosis D
  - Fanconi syndrome: Decrease in reabsorption of phosphate from the glomerular filtrate.
  - Physiological fall occurs whenever there is increased carbohydrate utilization, e.g., in the treatment of diabetic coma by injection of insulin. Insulin enhances transport of phosphate from extracellular fluid into the cells leading to fall in serum inorganic phosphate.

ASSESSMENT QUESTION

Q. Case-based quantitative estimation.
A 3-year-old boy with developmental delay presented with bowed legs, broad and tender wrists. The physician ordered serum calcium, vitamin D. The serum sample of the patient is provided to you. Identify the case and do the estimation of other relevant parameter. Express your result and interpret.

VIVA QUESTIONS

1. Which method is used to estimate serum phosphorus? Give its principle.
2. What is the normal range of serum phosphorus?
3. Name different conditions leading to hyperphosphatemia.
4. Name different conditions leading to hypophosphatemia.
5. What are the manifestations of hypophosphatemia?
6. What are the manifestations of hyperphosphatemia?
7. Renal failure causes hyperphosphatemia. Explain.

EXPERIMENT 26

Estimation of Serum Bilirubin

COMPETENCY	LEARNING OBJECTIVES
BI11.12: Demonstrate the estimation of serum bilirubin.	1. Perform estimation of serum bilirubin, interpret the results and give clinical significance.

INTRODUCTION

Bilirubin is an orange yellow bile pigment produced from the catabolism of heme of hemoprotein—hemoglobin, myoglobin, cytochromes and peroxidases. There are two types of bilirubin in the blood—**unconjugated (indirect) bilirubin** is insoluble in water and **conjugated (direct) bilirubin** is water soluble. Bilirubin is conjugated in the liver by glucuronate and excreted in bile.

Routine blood tests for total bilirubin measure both unconjugated and conjugated bilirubin. Any increase of bilirubin in blood is indicative of jaundice. The differentiation between the direct and indirect bilirubin is important in diagnosing the cause of hyperbilirubinemia.

ESTIMATION OF SERUM BILIRUBIN

Method: Malloy and Evelyn method
Specimen: Serum
Serum sample collection: Collect blood in a red-colored top vacutainer tube. Then allow the blood to clot the blood by leaving it undisturbed at room temperature for 15-6 minutes. Remove the clot by centrifuging at 1,000–2,000 RPM for 10 minutes. The resulting supernatant is serum.

Principle

This method is based on Van den Bergh's reaction in which bilirubin couples with diazotized sulfanilic acid to form a purple-colored azobilirubin. Conjugated/direct bilirubin which is water-soluble reacts with the diazo reagent in aqueous solution. The unconjugated/indirect bilirubin which is water insoluble is diazotized only in the presence of methanol. The subsequent addition of methanol accelerates the reaction of indirect bilirubin. Total bilirubin value (conjugated + unconjugated bilirubin) is obtained by direct and indirect reaction. The intensity of the color is directly proportional to the concentration of total bilirubin in the sample. The optical densities of colored solution are taken at 540 nm.

Reagents

- Diazo reagent (sulfanilic acid and sodium nitrite in HCL)
- Diazo blank reagent (1.5% HCl)
- Methanol
- Bilirubin standard in chloroform (0.1 mg/mL)

Procedure

Take six clean and dry test tubes and label them as given below and proceed as given in the **Table 26.1**.
1. S (standard)
2. B (blank)
3. DT (direct test)
4. DC (direct control)
5. TT (total test)
6. TC (total control)

Table 26.1: Procedure for serum bilirubin estimation.

Additions	Standard S	Blank B	Direct bilirubin DT	Direct bilirubin DC	Total bilirubin TT	Total bilirubin TC
Distilled water	1.8 mL	2 mL	4.3 mL	4.3 mL	1.8 mL	1.8 mL
Serum	-	-	0.2 mL	0.2 mL	0.2 mL	0.2 mL
Bilirubin std.	0.2 mL	-	-	-	-	-
Diazo color reagent	0.5 mL	0.5 mL	0.5 mL	-	0.5 mL	-
Diazo blank reagent (1.5% HCl)	-	-	-	0.5 mL	-	0.5 mL
Methanol	2.5 mL	2.5 mL	-	-	2.5 mL	2.5 mL

Mix, keep the tubes for 6 minutes in dark and read OD colorimetrically at 530 nm/green filter.

Observations

OD B
OD S
OD DC
OD DT
OD TC
OD TT

Calculations

a. **Direct bilirubin** (mg/dL)

$$= \frac{OD\ DT - ODC}{OD\ S - OD\ B} \times \frac{Conc.\ of\ std.}{Vol.\ of\ sample} \times 100$$

$$= \frac{OD\ DT - ODC}{OD\ S - OD\ B} \times \frac{0.02}{0.2} \times 100$$

$$= \frac{OD\ DT - ODC}{OD\ S - OD\ B} \times 10$$

= _____ mg/dL

b. **Total bilirubin** (mg/dL) $= \dfrac{\text{OD DT-OTC}}{\text{OD S-OD B}} \times \dfrac{\text{Conc. of std.}}{\text{Vol. of sample}} \times 100$

$= \dfrac{\text{OD DT-OTC}}{\text{OD S-OD B}} \times 10$

= _____ mg/dL.

c. **Unconjugated bilirubin** (mg/dL) = Total bilirubin (mg/dL) − Conjugated bilirubin (mg/dL)
= _____ mg/dL

Results

Conjugated bilirubin = _____ mg/dL
Unconjugated bilirubin = _____ mg/dL
Total bilirubin = _____ mg/dL

Normal Reference Range

Serum total bilirubin: 0.1–1.0 mg/dL
Serum conjugated (direct) bilirubin: 0.1–0.4 mg/dL
Serum unconjugated (indirect) bilirubin: 0.2–0.7 mg/dL

Other Method

Modified **Jendrassik and Gorf's** method

In this method, caffeine-benzoate reagent is used as an accelelator and an alkaline tartarate reagent is added after the reaction to form blue-green azobilirubin that is measured at 600 nm.

Clinical Significance

Elevated level of bilirubin in blood is known as 'hyperbilirubinemia'. Elevated levels of bilirubin are found in:
❖ Liver diseases (hepatitis, cirrhosis)
❖ Excessive hemolysis/destruction of RBCs (hemolytic jaundice)
❖ Obstruction to biliary track (obstructive jaundice)
❖ Drug-induced reactions

In hemolytic jaundice, the unconjugated fraction rises, whereas in hepatotoxic and obstructive jaundice, conjugated fraction is high. Based on the increased levels of conjugated and unconjugated bilirubin, the conditions can be classified as conjugated (direct) hyperbilirubinemia and unconjugated (indirect) hyperbilirubinemia.

ASSESSMENT QUESTION

Q. Case-based quantitative estimation.
A 15-year-old girl was admitted to the medical ward with the symptoms:
❖ Yellowish discoloration of the eye,
❖ Marked loss of appetite,
❖ Low grade fever,
❖ Nausea and occasional vomiting in the last one week,
❖ Pain in the right hypochondrium and
❖ Dark-colored urine
❖ Significant increased level of ALP

Identify the case and do the estimation of relevant parameter. Express your result and interpret.

VIVA QUESTIONS

1. What is bilirubin and how it is formed?
2. What is direct and indirect bilirubin?
3. Which method used for the estimation of bilirubin?
4. What is the other method for bilirubin estimation?
5. What is the principle of bilirubin estimation?
6. What are the normal ranges of total, direct and indirect bilirubin?
7. What is hyperbilirubinemia?
8. What are the common types of jaundice?

EXPERIMENT 27

Estimation of Serum Transaminases (SGPT/ALT and SGOT/AST)

COMPETENCY	LEARNING OBJECTIVES
BI11.13 Demonstrate the estimation of SGOT/SGPT.	1. Perform estimation of serum alanine transaminase (ALT), interpret the results and give clinical significance. 2. Perform estimation of serum aspartate transaminase (AST), interpret the results and give clinical significance.

INTRODUCTION

Aspartate transaminase (AST) and alanine transaminase (ALT) are the two clinically important enzymes catalyzing transfer of amino group from an alpha amino acid to an alpha keto acid. ALT is found predominantly in the liver, with clinically negligible quantities found in the kidneys, heart, and skeletal muscle, while AST is found in the liver, heart (cardiac muscle), skeletal muscle, kidneys, brain, and red blood cells.

❖ Alanine transaminase (ALT) is also called serum glutamate-pyruvate transaminase (SGPT) catalyze the following reaction:

$$\text{L-alanine} + \alpha\text{-ketoglutarate} \xrightleftharpoons[\text{PLP}]{\text{ALT or GPT}} \text{Pyruvate} + \text{L-glutamate}$$

❖ Aspartate transaminase (AST) is also called serum glutamate-oxaloacetate transaminase (SGOT) catalyze the following reaction:

$$\text{L-aspartate} + \alpha\text{-ketoglutarate} \xrightleftharpoons[\text{PLP}]{\text{AST or GOT}} \text{Oxaloacetate} + \text{L-glutamate}$$

The activities of ALT (SGPT) and AST (SGOT) are determined by measuring the keto acids produced, i.e., pyruvate for ALT and oxaloacetate for AST.

ESTIMATION OF SERUM ALANINE TRANSAMINASE (ALT)

Method used: Reitman & Frankel's method (Chemical colorimetric method)
Specimen: Serum
Serum sample collection: Collect blood in a red-colored top vacutainer tube. Then allow the blood to clot the blood by leaving it undisturbed at room temperature for 15–6 minutes. Remove the clot by centrifuging at 1,000–2,000 RPM for 10 minutes. The resulting supernatant is serum.

Principle

Transaminases are the enzymes catalyzing transfer of amino group from an alpha amino acid to an alpha keto acid. ALT in serum catalyzes the transfer of amino group from alanine to α-ketoglutarate yielding L-glutamate and pyruvate (keto acid). The keto acid pyruvate is treated with 2,4-dinitrophenyl hydrazine (DNPH) in alkaline medium to form reddish – brown complex of hydrazones. The intensity of the color is proportional to the amount of pyruvate present which in turn is proportional to the amount of ALT present in serum. Thus a measure of optical density of the colored solution indicates the concentration of the serum ALT. The optical density of color is read colorimetrically at 530 nm and compared with that of a standard pyruvate solution treated similarly. The activity of transaminase is expressed as international units (IU) and is defined as number of micromoles of respective keto acids formed per min per liter of serum.

Reagents

- Phosphate buffer: 0.1 M pH 7.4
- Standard pyruvic acid solution: (0.2 mg/mL = 2 mmol/mL)
- Substrate: L- alanine + α-ketoglutarate
- 2,4-dinitrophenyl hydrazine (DNPH) reagent
- 0.4 N NaOH

Procedure

Take clean and dry test tubes and label them as Blank (B), Standard (S) and 'Test (T) and proceed as given in the **Table 27.1**.

Table 27.1: Procedure for serum alanine transaminase (ALT).

Reagents	Blank (B)	Standard (S)	Control (C)	Test (T)
Substrate (Aspartate + α-ketoglutarate)	0.6 mL	0.5 mL	0.5 mL	0.5 mL
Standard (Pyruvic acid)	-	0.1 mL	-	-
Serum	-	-	-	0.1 mL
Incubate at 37°C for 30 minutes for ALT				
DNPH	0.5 mL	0.5 mL	0.5 mL	0.5 mL
Serum	-	-	0.1 mL	-
Allow to stand for 20 minutes at room temperature				
0.4 N NaOH	5 mL	5 mL	5 mL	5 mL

Mix and keep at RT for 10 minutes. Read optical density using colorimeter at 530 nm/green filter.

Observations

OD B
OD S
OD C
OD T

ESTIMATION OF SERUM ASPARTATE TRANSAMINASE (AST)

Method used: Reitman & Frankel's method (Chemical colorimetric method)
Specimen: Serum
Serum sample collection: Collect blood in a red-colored top vacutainer tube. Then allow the blood to clot the blood by leaving it undisturbed at room temperature for 15–6 minutes. Remove the clot by centrifuging at 1,000–2,000 RPM for 10 minutes. The resulting supernatant is serum.

EXPERIMENT 27: Estimation of Serum Transaminases (SGPT/ALT and SGOT/AST)

Principle

Transaminases are the enzymes catalyzing transfer of amino group from an alpha amino acid to an alpha keto acid. AST in serum catalyzes the transfer of amino group from aspartate to α-ketoglutarate yielding L-glutamate and oxaloacetate (keto acid). The keto acid oxaloacetate is treated with 2,4-dinitrophenyl hydrazine (DNPH) in alkaline medium to form reddish–brown complex of hydrazones. The intensity of the color is proportional to the amount of oxaloacetate present which in turn is proportional to the amount of AST present in serum. Thus a measure of optical density of the colored solution indicates the concentration of the serum AST. The optical density of color is read colorimetrically at 530 nm and compared with that of a standard oxaloacetate solution treated similarly.

Reagents

1. Phosphate buffer: 0.1M pH 7.4
2. Standard oxaloacetic acid solution: (0.2 mg/mL = 2 mmol/mL)
3. Substrate: L- aspartate + α-ketoglutarate
4. 2,4-dinitrophenyl hydrazine (DNPH)
5. 0.4 N NaOH

Procedure

Take clean and dry test tubes and label them as Blank (B), Standard (S) and 'Test (T) and proceed as given in the **Table 27.2**.

Table 27.2: Procedure for serum aspartate transaminase (AST).

Reagents	Blank (B)	Standard (S)	Control (C)	Test (T)
Substrate (Aspartate + α-ketoglutarate)	0.6 mL	0.5 mL	0.5 mL	0.5 mL
Standard (oxaloacetic acid)	-	0.1 mL	-	-
Serum	-	-	-	0.1 mL
Incubate at 37°C for 60 minutes				
DNPH	0.5 mL	0.5 mL	0.5 mL	0.5 mL
Serum	-	-	0.1 mL	-
Allow to stand for 20 minutes at room temperature				
0.4 N NaOH	5 mL	5 mL	5 mL	5 mL

Mix and keep at RT for 10 minutes. Read optical density using colorimeter at 530 nm/green filter.

Observations

OD B
OD S
OD C
OD T

Calculations

Activity of transaminase is expressed in terms of international units. International unit is defined as micromoles of pyruvate formed at 37°C in one minute by enzyme activity present in 1000 mL of serum.

ALT activity (IU/L) $= \dfrac{OD\ T - OD\ C}{OD\ S - OD\ B} \times 66.66$

$= \underline{\hspace{2cm}}$ IU/L

AST activity (IU/L) $= \dfrac{OD\ T - OD\ C}{OD\ S - OD\ B} \times 33.33$

$= \underline{\hspace{2cm}}$ IU/L

Result

ALT activity = _____ IU/L
AST activity = _____ IU/L

Normal Reference Range

- **Activity of ALT:** 5–40 IU/L
- **Activity of AST:** 5–35 IU/L

Clinical Significance

Highest activity of AST is in the myocardium and next in the liver and next in skeletal muscle. However highest activity of ALT is in the liver. The concentration of ALT in heart muscle is only a fraction of that of AST activity. In clinical practice, both AST and ALT are assayed for diagnosing liver disease and AST is used for evaluating ischemic heart disease.
- Both plasma AST and ALT levels are elevated in liver disease
- Although serum levels of both AST and ALT become elevated in liver diseases, ALT is the more liver specific enzyme.
- ALT is an early and specific indicator of hepatic diseases. The enzyme activity rises before clinical signs appear or serum bilirubin starts rising.
- Plasma ALT elevations are rarely observed in conditions other than liver disease.
- Increased AST level occurs after myocardial infarction as heart muscles contain relatively high concentration of AST.
- After acute myocardial infarction, AST activity increases. The enzyme activity starts rising only after 6 to 8 hours after the onset of chest pain and it peaks around 18–24 hours and falls within the normal range by the fourth or fifth day, provided no new infarct has occurred.
- Raised AST activity is also observed in hepatocellular damage, e.g., due to hepatotoxic drug, infective hepatitis, primary or secondary liver cancer, but rise in AST activity in these condition is much less significant than ALT activity.
- AST and occasionally ALT levels are increased in muscular dystrophy.

ASSESSMENT QUESTIONS

Q1. Case-based quantitative estimation.
A 20-year-old girl staying in a college hostel brought to the outpatient clinic of medical college with complaints of fever, headache, nausea and yellowish discoloration of sclera. Following are the results of the tests:
- Level of ALP is found to be normal
- Increased level of conjugated and unconjugated bilirubin is found

Identify the case and do the estimation of relevant enzyme. Express your result and interpret.

Q2. Case-based quantitative estimation.
A 66-year-old man sought medical care at the hospital due to severe chest pain lasting for 12 hours. The patient was aware of being hypertensive and was a smoker. Without any prior symptom, he started to have severe chest pain and sought emergency medical care after about 12 hours, due to pain persistence. Identify the case and do the estimation of relevant enzyme. Express your result and interpret.

VIVA QUESTIONS

1. What are the normal blood levels of SGPT and SGOT?
2. Which tissues have the maximum concentration of SGPT and SGOT?
3. What is the clinical significance of SGPT (ALT) estimations?
4. Give the principle of a method employed in the assay of SGPT and SGOT.
5. What is the clinical significance of SGOT (AST) estimations?

EXPERIMENT 28

Estimation of Serum Alkaline Phosphatase

COMPETENCY	LEARNING OBJECTIVES
BI11.14 Demonstrate the estimation of alkaline phosphatase.	1. Perform estimation of serum alkaline phosphatase, interpret the results and give clinical significance.

INTRODUCTION

Alkaline phosphatase (ALP) is an enzyme that catalyzes hydrolysis of phosphate ester to liberate phosphoric acid at alkaline pH (pH of 10). ALP exists as several isoenzymes which are found in high concentrations in the liver, bone, intestine, kidney and placenta. Damage to these tissues causes the release of ALP into the blood. Alkaline phosphatase activity is important for the mineralization of bone and represents a useful biochemical marker of bone formation. Growing children have higher levels of alkaline phosphatase than full-grown adults due to increased osteoblast activity following accelerated bone growth.

ESTIMATION OF SERUM ALKALINE PHOSPHATASE

Method used: Kind and King's method
Specimen: Serum
Serum sample collection: Collect blood in a red-colored top vacutainer tube. Then allow the blood to clot the blood by leaving it undisturbed at room temperature for 15–6 minutes. Remove the clot by centrifuging at 1,000–2,000 RPM for 10 minutes. The resulting supernatant is serum.

Principle

ALP at pH around 10 hydrolyses disodium phenyl phosphate to form phenol phosphoric acid. The phenol formed reacts with 4-aminoantipyrine in the presence of alkaline oxidizing agent potassium ferricyanide to give purple color. The intensity of color developed is a measure of enzyme activity and is read colorimetrically at 530 nm.

Reagents

- **Bicarbonate buffer (pH 10):** Sodium carbonate-sodium bicarbonate
- **Substrate:** Disodium phenyl phosphate

- 0.5N NaOH
- 0.5N Na_2CO_3
- 4-Aminoantipyrine
- Potassium ferricyanide
- **Phenol standard concentration:** 0.01 mg/mL = 10/94 micromoles/mL = 0.106 mmol/mL

Procedure

Take clean and dry test tubes and label them as Blank (B), Standard (S) and 'Test (T) and proceed as given in the **Table 28.1.**

Table 28.1: Procedure for serum alkaline phosphatase (ALP).

Reagents	Blank (B)	Standard (S)	Control (C)	Test (T)
	1.0 mL Distilled water	1.0 mL Standard phenol solution	1.0 mL Bicarbonate buffer	1.0 mL Bicarbonate buffer
Substrate (Disodium phenyl phosphate)	1.1 mL	1.1 mL	1.0 mL	1.0 mL
Serum	--	--	--	0.1 mL
Mix I and incubate at 37°C for 15 minutes				
0.5N NaOH	0.8 mL	0.8 mL	0.8 mL	0.8 mL
0.5N Na_2CO_3	1.2 mL	1.2 mL	1.2 mL	1.2 mL
Serum	--	--	0.1 mL	--
4-Aminoantipyrine	1.0 mL	1.0 mL	1.0 mL	1.0 mL
Potassium ferricyanide	1.0 mL	1.0 mL	1.0 mL	1.0 mL

Mix after each addition. Read colorimetrically at 530 nm/green filter immediately.

Observations

OD B

OD S

OD C

OD T

Calculations

Serum alkaline phosphatase activity is expressed in terms of King Armstrong units (KA units) and international units (IU/L)

- **King Armstrong units (KA units):** KA units are defined as mg of phenol liberated by enzyme activity present in 100 mL of serum at 37°C in 15 minutes.

- **ALP activity** (KA units) $= \dfrac{OD\ T - ODC}{OD\ S - OD\ B} \times 10$

  = _____ KA units

- **International units (IU/L):** IU/L is defined as micromoles of phenol liberated by enzyme activity present in 1000 mL of serum at 37°C in 1 minute.

  ALP activity (IU/L) $= \dfrac{OD\ T - ODC}{OD\ S - OD\ B} \times 71$

  = _____ IU/L

Result

ALP activity = _____ KA units

ALP activity = _____ IU/L

Normal Reference Values

ALP activity: 3–13 KA units
ALP activity: 23–92 IU/L

Other Methods

- King and Armstrong,
- Bowers and McComb method

Clinical Significance

- Increased levels are associated mainly with liver and bone disease. Serum ALP measurements are of particular interest in the investigation of hepatobiliary disease and bone disease.
- A rise in the alkaline phosphatase occurs with all forms of cholestasis, particularly with obstructive jaundice.
- An increased serum alkaline phosphatase may be due to obstruction of the biliary tract. When the liver, bile ducts or gallbladder system are not functioning properly or are blocked, this enzyme is not excreted through the bile and alkaline phosphatase is released into the blood stream.
- In addition to liver, bile duct, or gallbladder dysfunction, an elevated serum alkaline phosphatase can be due to rapid growth of bone since it is produced by bone-forming cells called osteoblasts.
- It is also elevated in diseases of the skeletal system, such as Paget disease, hyperparathyroidism, rickets and osteomalacia, as well as with fractures and malignant tumors.

ASSESSMENT QUESTION

Q. Case-based quantitative estimation.
A 55-year-old woman having pain in the upper right side of the abdomen, fever with chills, pruritus (severe itching of the skin) and passing dark urine and clay colored stools. Increased level of conjugated bilirubin is also found. The physician asked for enzyme analysis. Identify the case and do the estimation of relevant parameter. Express your result and interpret.

VIVA QUESTIONS

1. What is the optimum pH of alkaline phosphates?
2. What are the normal blood levels of serum alkaline phosphatase?
3. What is the role of alkaline phosphatase in the diagnosis of jaundice?
4. Name conditions other than liver disease where estimating serum alkaline phosphatase is useful.
5. Name various isoenzymes of alkaline phosphatase.

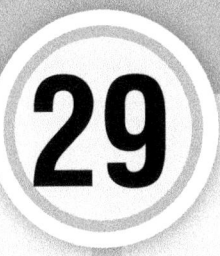

EXPERIMENT 29

Estimation of Serum Total Cholesterol

COMPETENCY	LEARNING OBJECTIVES
BI11.9 Demonstrate estimation of serum cholesterol and HDL cholesterol.	1. Perform estimation of serum total cholesterol interpret the result and give clinical significance.

INTRODUCTION

Cholesterol is the main lipid found in blood, bile and brain tissues. Cholesterol is present exclusively in animal derived foods. It is required for the formation of steroids and cellular membranes and is essential for nerve impulse conduction.

Cholesterol is transported in the form of low density lipoprotein (LDL), and high density lipoprotein (HDL).
- LDL carries cholesterol to the peripheral tissues where it can be deposited and increase the risk of arteriosclerotic heart and peripheral vascular disease. Hence, high levels of LDL are atherogenic. This is the reason LDL cholesterol is called *'bad cholesterol.'*
- HDL transport cholesterol from the peripheral tissues to the liver for excretion, hence HDL cholesterol has a protective effect. This is the reason HDL cholesterol is called *'good cholesterol.'*

ESTIMATION OF SERUM TOTAL CHOLESTEROL

Method used: Chemical method: Zak's method
Specimen: Serum
Serum sample collection: Collect whole blood after 9–12 hours fasting in a red color-coded vacuum evacuated tube. After collection of the whole blood, allow the blood to clot by leaving it undisturbed at room temperature for 30 minutes. Remove the clot by centrifuging at 1,000–2,000 RPM for 10 minutes. The resulting supernatant is serum.

Principle

Proteins in serum are precipitated by ferric chloride–acetic acid reagent. The cholesterol present in protein free filtrate (PFF) is oxidized and dehydrated with ferric chloride, acetic acid and sulfuric acid to a red colored compound. The intensity of color produced is directly proportional to the concentration of total cholesterol present in the sample measured at 540 nm.

Reagents

- **Ferric chloride:** Acetic acid reagent (0.05 g ferric chloride +100 mL of acetic acid)
- Conc. H_2SO_4
- Stock cholesterol standard solution (100 mg cholesterol in 100 mL acetic acid)
- **Working cholesterol standard (0.04 mg/mL):** Dilute 1 mL stock cholesterol to 25 mL with ferric chloride acetic acid reagent.

Procedure

- **Part I: Preparation of protein free filtrate (PFF)**—in a dry centrifuge test tube, take 9.8 mL of ferric chloride/acetic acid reagent and 0.2 mL serum. Cover the mouth with a piece of paraffin film and mix by inversion. Keep for 15 minutes for the proteins to precipitate. Centrifuge and use clear supernatant as PFF.
- **Part II:** Take clean and dry test tubes and label them as Blank (B), Standard (S) and 'Test (T) and proceed as given in the **Table 29.1**.

Table 29.1: Procedure for serum total cholesterol.

Reagents	Blank (B)	Standard (S)	Test (T)
	5 mL $FeCl_3$; acetic acid reagent	5 mL Std. cholesterol	5 mL PFF
Conc. H_2SO_4	3 mL	3 mL	3 mL

Mix by swirling slowly, keep for 6 minutes, and read OD using colorimeter at 540 nm.

Observations

OD B
OD S
OD T

Calculations

Serum total cholesterol (mg /dL)

$$= \frac{OD\ T - OD\ B}{OD\ S - OD\ .B} \times \frac{Conc.\ of\ std.}{Vol.\ of\ sample} \times 100$$

$$= \frac{OD\ T - OD\ B}{OD\ S - OD\ .B} \times \frac{0.02}{0.1} \times 100$$

$$= \frac{OD\ T - OD\ B}{OD\ S - OD\ B} \times 200$$

= _____ mg/dL

Result

Total cholesterol = _____ mg/dL

Normal Reference Range

<200 mg/dL

Other Method

Cholesterol oxidase: Peroxidase (CHOD-PAP) enzymatic kit method
The series of reactions involved in this assay system are:
- Cholesterol esterase hydrolyses cholesterol ester to free cholesterol.
- Free cholesterol is then oxidized by cholesterol oxidase (CHOD).
- In this reaction, hydrogen peroxide is produced as a byproduct. From hydrogen peroxide nascent oxygen is produced by the catalytic action of peroxidase (POD).
- Nascent oxygen then reacts with phenol and 4-aminoantipyrine to form a red-colored quinoneimine complex. The OD of which measured colorimetrically at 56 nm. Intensity of color formed is directly proportional to the amount of cholesterol present in the sample.

Clinical Significance

- Desirable level suggested by National Cholesterol Education Program (NCEP) to total cholesterol is:
  - Adult <200 mg%
  - Children and adolescent <170 mg%
- **Hypercholesterolemia is very common** and associated with an increased risk of CHD. Hypercholesterolemia is seen in:
  - Diabetes mellitus
  - Nephrotic syndrome
  - Obstructive jaundice
  - Hypothyroidism
  - Xanthomatosis
- **Hypocholesterolemia is uncommon**. It is observed in:
  - Hyperthyroidism,
  - Hemolytic jaundice
  - Malabsorption syndrome
  - Serum cholesterol concentration is very low in rare genetic disease, such as abetalipoproteinemia.

ASSESSMENT QUESTION

Q. Case-based quantitative estimation.
A 9-year-old boy came to the outpatient department with cutaneous xanthoma on the elbow and hands. His father had expired at the age of 35 years following a sudden heart attack. The serum sample of the patient is provided to you. Identify the case and do the estimation of relevant parameter. Express your result and interpret.

VIVA QUESTIONS

1. What is the importance of estimating blood cholesterol?
2. Desirable level suggested by National Cholesterol Education Program (NCEP) to total cholesterol.
3. Mention the principle of an enzymatic method for cholesterol estimation.
4. What are the major causes of hypercholesterolemia?
5. What are the major causes of hypocholesterolemia?

EXPERIMENT 30

Estimation of Serum HDL Cholesterol

COMPETENCY	LEARNING OBJECTIVES
BI11.9 Demonstrate estimation of serum cholesterol and HDL cholesterol.	1. Perform estimation of serum HDL cholesterol, interpret the result and give clinical significance.

INTRODUCTION

A high-density lipoprotein (HDL) test measures the level of good cholesterol in blood. HDL transport cholesterol from the peripheral tissues to the liver for excretion, hence HDL cholesterol has a protective effect. This is the reason HDL cholesterol is called **good cholesterol.**

ESTIMATION OF SERUM HDL CHOLESTEROL

Method used: Polyethylene glycol/Cholesterol oxidase-Peroxidase (PEG/CHOD-PAP) enzymatic method (Kit method)
Specimen: Serum
Serum sample collection: Collect whole blood after 9–12 hours fasting in a red color-coded vacuum evacuated tube. After collection of the whole blood, allow the blood to clot by leaving it undisturbed at room temperature for 30 minutes. Remove the clot by centrifuging at 1,000–2,000 RPM for 10 minutes. The resulting supernatant is serum.

Principle

Low density lipoprotein (LDL) cholesterol, very low density lipoproteins (VLDL) cholesterol and chylomicrons fractions are precipitated by addition of polyethylene glycol 6000 (PEG). After centrifugation, the high density lipoprotein (HDL) fraction remains in the supernatant and is determined with CHOD-PAP method. The absorbance of which measured colorimetrically at 530 nm. Intensity of color formed is directly proportional to the amount of HDL cholesterol present in the sample.

Reagents

- **Cholesterol reagent:** Containing cholesterol esterase, cholesterol oxidase, peroxidase, and 4-aminoantipyrine.
- **Precipitating reagent:** Polyethylene glycol 6000 (PEG)
- HDL cholesterol standard (50 mg/dL)

Procedure (Table 30.1)

❖ **Separation of serum HDL cholesterol by precipitation of VLDL and LDL:** Pipette into a clean dry test tube take 0.1 mL of serum sample add to it 0.1 mL of precipitating reagent (PEG 6000). Mix well and keep at room temperature for 10 minutes then centrifuge at 2000 rpm for 10 minutes to obtain a clear supernatant. Use the supernatant for HDL cholesterol estimation.

❖ Take clean and dry test tubes and label them as Blank (B), Standard (S) and 'Test (T) and proceed as given in the **Table 30.1**.

Table 30.1: Procedure for serum HDL cholesterol.

Reagents	Blank (B)	Standard (S)	Test (T)
Cholesterol working reagent	1.0 mL	1.0 mL	1.0 mL
Distilled water	0.01 mL	—	—
HDL cholesterol std.	—	0.01 mL	—
Supernatant from step 1	—	—	0.01 mL

Mix well and incubate at 37°C for 10 minutes. Read colorimetrically at 530 nm/green filter.

Observations

OD S
OD T
OD B

Calculations

HDL cholesterol (mg /dL) $= \dfrac{OD\ T - OD\ B}{OD\ S - OD\ B} \times 25 \times 2$ (dilution factor)

= _____ mg/dL

Results

HDL cholesterol   = _____ mg/dL

Normal Reference Range

	HDL cholesterol
Normal	Men: 6–60 mg/dL Women: 40–70 mg/dL
High risk	<40 mg/dL
Low risk	≥60 mg/dL

Clinical Significance

The measurement of total and HDL cholesterol provide valuable information for the risk assessment of coronary heart diseases (CHD).

❖ Increased HDL cholesterol concentration reduces the risk of cardiovascular disease. HDL transport cholesterol from the peripheral tissues to the liver for excretion, hence HDL cholesterol has a protective effect.

❖ Decreased HDL cholesterol concentration increases the risk of CHD. It is lowered in Tangier disease, cigarette smoking, obesity, very high carbohydrate diets, and uncontrolled diabetes mellitus and in male sex hormone therapy.

VIVA QUESTIONS

1. Give the principle of enzymatic method of HDL cholesterol estimation.
2. What is the clinical significance of HDL?
3. What is the normal HDL level?
4. Why HDL cholesterol called good cholesterol?

EXPERIMENT 31

Estimation of Serum Triglycerides

COMPETENCY	LEARNING OBJECTIVES
BI11.10 Demonstrate the estimation of triglycerides.	1. Perform estimation of triglycerides interpret the result and give clinical significance.

INTRODUCTION

A triglyceride (TG) or triacylglycerol (TAG) consisting of three fatty acids esterified to a glycerol backbone. Triglycerides are the main storage form of fat in humans and acts as a storage source of energy. Triglycerides are transported in the blood as lipoproteins. Chylomicrons and VLDL are rich in TG content.

ESTIMATION OF SERUM TRIGLYCERIDES

Method: Enzymatic method: Glycerol phosphate oxidase-Peroxidase (GPO-PAP) enzymatic method.
Specimen: Serum
Serum sample collection: Collect whole blood after 9–12 hours fasting in a red color-coded vacuum evacuated tube. After collection of the whole blood, allow the blood to clot by leaving it undisturbed at room temperature for 30 minutes. Remove the clot by centrifuging at 1,000–2,000 RPM for 10 minutes. The resulting supernatant is serum.

Principle

Lipoprotein lipase hydrolyses triglycerides to glycerol and free fatty acids. The glycerol formed reacts with ATP in the presence of glycerol kinase to form glycerol 3-phosphate. Glycerol 3-phosphate is oxidized by the enzyme glycerol phosphate oxidase to dihydroxyacetone phosphate and hydrogen peroxide. The hydrogen peroxide further reacts with 4-aminoantipyrine by the catalytic action of peroxidase to form a pink-colored quinoneimine. The intensity of which measured colorimetrically at 530 nm. Intensity of color formed is directly proportional to the amount of TG present in the sample.

Reagents

Readymade kits are available which contain:
- Triglyceride enzyme reagents
- Triglyceride Standard (200 mg/dL)

Procedure

Take clean and dry test tubes and label them as Blank (B), Standard (S) and 'Test (T) and proceed as given in the **Table 31.1**.

Table 31.1: Procedure for serum triglyceride.

Reagents	Blank (B)	Standard (S)	Test (T)
Working enzyme reagent	1.0 mL	1.0 mL	1.0 mL
Distilled water	10 µL	--	--
Triglyceride standard	--	10 µL	--
Serum sample	--	--	10 µL

Mix and incubate at 37°C for 10 minutes. Read colorimetrically at 530 nm/green filter.

Observations

OD S

OD T

OD B

Calculations

Triglycerides (mg/dL) $= \dfrac{\text{OD T}}{\text{OD S}} \times 200$

= _____ mg/dL

Normal Reference Range

	Triglycerides mg/dL
Normal range	<150
Borderline	150–200
High risk	200–500
Very high risk	500 or higher

Clinical Significance

❖ The measurement of TG levels is useful in the diagnosis of primary and secondary hyperlipoproteinemia, dyslipidemia, and triglyceridemia.
❖ TG concentrations are also useful in the diagnosis and treatment of diabetes mellitus, nephrosis, liver obstruction and other diseases involving lipid metabolism or various endocrine disorders.
❖ High levels of triglycerides are associated with atherosclerosis, heart disease and stroke. The risk can be partly accounted for by a strong inverse relationship between triglyceride level and HDL-cholesterol level.
❖ A triglyceride level <150 mg/dL is considered ideal for adults, according to the guidelines of National Cholesterol Education Program. A triglyceride level of 150 to 200 mg/dL is borderline high. A triglyceride result of 200 to 500 mg/dL is high, and levels of 500 mg/dL or more are very high.

ASSESSMENT QUESTION

Q. Case-based quantitative estimation.

A-52-year-old project manager in an IT company have heart problem came for hospital. He was known diabetic for last 15 years neglecting physical exercise. After examining, the physician ordered lipid profile (total cholesterol, HDL-C ,

LDL-C). The serum sample of the patient is provided to you. Identify the case and do the estimation of remaining relevant parameter of lipid profile. Express your result and interpret.

VIVA QUESTIONS

1. Which method is used for estimation of triglycerides?
2. What is the normal level of triglycerides in the blood?
3. What is the clinical importance of estimating serum triacylglycerols?
4. What are the common causes of hypertriglyceridemia?

SECTION D
Basis and Rationale of Biochemical Tests Done in Various Disorders (SGD)

Section Outline

Experiment 32: Basis and Rationale of Biochemical Tests Done in Various Disorders

EXPERIMENT 32

Basis and Rationale of Biochemical Tests Done in Various Disorders

COMPETENCY	LEARNING OBJECTIVES
BI11.17 Explain the basis and rationale of biochemical tests done in the following conditions: Diabetes mellitus, dyslipidemia, myocardial infarction, renal failure, gout, proteinuria, nephrotic syndrome, edema, jaundice, liver diseases, pancreatitis, disorders of acid-base balance, thyroid disorders.	1. Describe the basis and rationale of biochemical tests done in: » Diabetes mellitus » Dyslipidemia » Myocardial infarction » Liver disease, jaundice » Pancreatitis » Nephrotic syndrome » Renal failure » Proteinuria and edema » Gout » Thyroid disorders » Disorders of acid base balance

▋INTRODUCTION

Diagnostic tests performed in clinical laboratory can be used for diagnosis of disorder or risk assessment purposes or to assess a patient's response to treatments, or even to guide the selection of further tests and treatments. Diagnostic tests are also increasingly used to assess the quality of patient care that is provided for medical conditions, such as **diabetes**, **heart failure**, **liver disorders** and **colon cancer**.

▋BASIS AND RATIONALE OF BIOCHEMICAL TESTS DONE IN DIABETES MELLITUS (TABLE 32.1)

Diabetes mellitus is a metabolic disease characterized by hyperglycemia, caused by inherited and/or acquired defects in insulin secretion, insulin action, or both. The chronic hyperglycemia of diabetes is associated with long-term damage, dysfunction, and failure of different organs, especially the eyes, kidneys, nerves, heart, and blood vessels. The following investigations are helpful in diagnosis of diabetes mellitus:

❖ Urine testing
❖ Blood glucose estimation
❖ Glycated hemoglobin estimation

Table 32.1: Basis and rationale of biochemical tests done in diabetes mellitus.

No.	Biochemical tests	Basis/Rationale
1.	Urine testing	
	• Benedict's test for glucose	• Glucose is not normally found in urine, but it can pass from the kidneys into the urine in diabetes mellitus; when the blood glucose level exceeds renal threshold for glucose (180 mg/dL). The diagnosis of symptomatic cases of diabetes can be confirmed by glycosuria
	• Rothera's test for ketones	• During uncontrolled diabetes, the ketone bodies are synthesized within the liver. Poorly controlled diabetes mellitus is the most common pathologic condition causing ketonuria
2.	Blood glucose	• In symptomatic cases, the diagnosis can be confirmed by finding **blood glucose** level » Random blood sugar level of 200 mg/dL or higher suggests diabetes » Fasting blood sugar level less than 100 mg/dL is normal » A fasting blood sugar level from 100 to 125 mg/dL is considered prediabetes. If it is 126 mg/dL or higher is considered diabetes • Blood glucose testing also provides useful information for diabetes management
3.	Glycated hemoglobin (HbA1c)	• All above tests provide information about the patient's glucose concentration only at that time and may be unrepresentative of overall control • HbA1c is an important indicator of long-term glycemic control over the past 2 to 3 months and is a reliable biomarker for the diagnosis and prognosis of diabetes • HbA1c not only provides a reliable measure of chronic hyperglycemia but also correlates well with the risk of long-term diabetes complications • Elevated HbA1c has also been regarded as an independent risk factor for coronary heart disease and stroke in subjects with/without diabetes

BASIS AND RATIONALE OF BIOCHEMICAL TESTS DONE IN DYSLIPIDEMIA (TABLE 32.2)

❖ Disorders of lipoprotein metabolism are collectively referred to as "dyslipidemias." Dyslipidemias are generally characterized clinically by increased plasma levels of cholesterol, triglycerides, low density lipoprotein (LDL), variably accompanied by reduced levels of high density lipoprotein (HDL). Dyslipidemias are associated with atherosclerosis, resulting in risk of cardiovascular disease (CVD).

❖ Dyslipidemias associated with lipoprotein metabolism due to different genetic causes are termed as **primary dyslipidemias** and dyslipidemias associated with other conditions, such as type 2 diabetes, obesity, alcoholism, hypothyroidism, or renal failure are termed **secondary dyslipidemias.**

Table 32.2: Basis and rationale of biochemical tests done in dyslipidemia.

No.	Biochemical Tests	Basis/Rationale
	Lipid profile tests (carried out in a fasting blood specimen)	
1.	Total serum cholesterol	• Unfortunately, high **cholesterol** does not cause symptoms but increased plasma levels of cholesterol are associated with atherosclerosis, resulting in risk of cardiovascular disease (CVD). » High risk: 240 mg/dL and above » Borderline high risk: 200–239 mg/dL » Desirable: <200 mg/dL
2.	LDL cholesterol	• **Low-density lipoprotein (LDL)** is the "bad cholesterol," the main cause of plaque build-up, which increases risk for heart disease. » High risk: 160 mg/dL and above » Borderline high risk: 100–159 mg/dL » Desirable: <100 mg/dL
3.	HDL cholesterol	• **High-density lipoproteins (HDL).** This is the "good cholesterol." It transports bad cholesterol from the blood to the liver, where it is excreted by the body. » High risk: <40 mg/dL for men and <50 mg/dL for women
4.	Serum triglycerides	• **Serum triglycerides** are also linked to heart disease. » Very high risk: 500 mg/dL and above » High risk: 200–499 mg/dL » Borderline high risk: 150–199 mg/dL » Normal: <150 mg/dL

- A **lipid profile** tests are used to identify the symptoms associated with dyslipidemia or abnormal levels of lipid and to estimate increased risk of cardiovascular disease. Lipid profile tests includes measurement of:
  - Total serum cholesterol (normal <200 mg/dL)
  - Serum triglycerides (normal 10 to 150 mg/dL)
  - HDL cholesterol (normal 40 to 60 mg/dL)
  - LDL cholesterol (normal 70 to 100 mg/dL)

BASIS AND RATIONALE OF BIOCHEMICAL TESTS DONE IN MYOCARDIAL INFARCTION (TABLE 32.3)

Myocardial infarction (MI) is a condition in which there is a rapid development of myocardial necrosis (cell or tissue death) due to an inadequate supply of blood and oxygen (ischemia) to a portion of the myocardium. The underlying pathology in MI is **atherosclerosis**, which cause narrowing of the arterial lumen, resulting in reduced myocardial oxygen supply.

The clinical manifestation of which is chest pain (angina pectoris). Pain characteristically involving the central portion of the chest and/or the epigastrium (upper part of abdomen), or radiating to left arm is the most common presenting complaint in patients with MI. Other signs may include breathlessness, giddiness, and uneasiness, vomiting and sweating.

Cardiac Biomarkers

After myocardial infarction, a number of intracellular enzymes and proteins are released from the damaged cells **(Table 32.3)**. They have diagnostic importance and are called cardiac biomarkers. Cardiac markers are useful in the detection of acute myocardial infarction (AMI) or minor myocardial injury. The cardiac markers of diagnostic interest include:

- **Enzymes:**
  - Creatine kinase (CK)
  - Lactate dehydrogenase (LD)
  - Serum aspartate aminotransferase (AST) also called serum glutamate transaminase (SGOT).
- **Nonenzyme proteins:** Cardiac troponin T and I (cTnT and cTnI)

Table 32.3: Basis and rationale of biochemical tests done in myocardial infarction.

No.	Biochemical tests	Basis/Rationale
1.	Creatinine kinase (CK-MB)	• CK is the first enzyme to appear in serum in higher concentration after MI. • CK-MB isoenzyme is a more sensitive and specific test than total CK. CK–MB is found exclusively in the myocardium, elevated CK–MB levels in serum are highly specific and sensitive for myocardial cell injury. • CK-MB rises within 4–6 hours after onset of chest pain, peaks at 12–24 hours. and returns to normal levels within 2–3 days.
2.	AST (SGOT)	• The first biomarker used to aid in the diagnosis of acute MI was aspartate aminotransferase (AST). • It is much less specific indication of myocardial infarction than the rise in CK. • In current clinical practice, AST has fallen out of favor for diagnosing acute MI because it is not a specific marker for cardiac myocytes. AST levels in the blood also elevate in hepatic disease (hepatitis), pericarditis, pulmonary embolism, and shock. • AST begins to rise about 6 to 12 hours after MI and peaks at 24 to 48 hours and returns to baseline within 5 days after the infarct.
3.	Lactate dehydrogenase (LDH)	• Serum total LDH values become elevated at 12 to 18 hours after onset of symptoms, peaks at 48 to 72 hours and returns to normal after 6 to 10 days. • The LDH1 (heart specific) increase over LDH2 in serum after AMI (flipped pattern), in which the LDH1/LDH2 ratio becomes greater than 1. • The use of LDH and LDH isoenzymes for detection of AMI is declining rapidly because its levels can also increase in many other conditions.
4.	Troponins (cTnI and cTnT)	• Cardiac troponins I (cTnI) and T (cTnT) are specific and sensitive biomarkers of cardiac ischemia, and they are the preferred blood test in the evaluation of patients suspected to have acute MI. • The initial rise in cardiac troponins after MI occurs at about the same time as CK–MB and remains elevated for 1 to 2 weeks. This property enables early as well as late diagnosis. • Thus, clinical evidence has been shown that either cTnT or cTnI can be replaced CK-MB as the test of choice to rule in or rule out MI.

BASIS AND RATIONALE OF BIOCHEMICAL TESTS DONE IN LIVER DISEASE AND JAUNDICE

Liver disorders may be classified as:
1. **Hepatocellular disease:** Inflammatory disease of the liver is termed **hepatitis** and may be acute or chronic.
   - Viral infection causes acute hepatitis whereas cirrhosis is the result of chronic hepatitis and is characterized by fibrosis of the hepatic cells.
   - The term **hepatic failure** indicates a clinical condition in which the biochemical function of the liver is severely and potentially fatally compromised.
2. **Cholestatic disease:** Cholestasis is the clinical term for biliary obstruction, which may occur in the small bile ducts in the liver itself or in the large extrahepatic ducts.
3. **Jaundice:** Jaundice clinically obvious when plasma bilirubin concentration exceed 3 mg/dL. Hyperbilirubinemia is the result of an imbalance between its production and excretion. The causes of jaundice are classified as follows:
   - **Prehepatic:** An increased rate of bilirubin production exceeds normal excretory capacity of the liver or impaired hepatic uptake of bilirubin.
   - **Hepatic:** The normal load of bilirubin cannot be conjugated and/or excreted by damaged liver cells.
   - **Posthepatic:** The biliary flow is obstructed, so that conjugated bilirubin cannot be excreted into the intestine and is regurgitate into the systemic circulation.

Tests for Diagnosis of Liver Diseases

Liver diseases may be diagnosed by liver function tests (LFTs). These are a group of tests that help in diagnosis, assessing prognosis and monitoring therapy. Different test can give different information about hepatic dysfunction. This then allows the selection of further investigations, such as ultrasound, CT scanning, magnetic resonance spectroscopy, endoscopy and liver biopsy.

- The standard biochemical tests used in assessing hepatobiliary disease include serum **(Table 32.4)**:
  - Alanine aminotransferase (ALT)
  - Alkaline phosphatase (ALP)
  - Gamma- glutamyl transpeptidase (GGT)
  - Bilirubin
  - Albumin
  - Prothrombin time
- These biochemical investigations can assist in differentiating:
  - Acute hepatocellular damage
  - Obstruction to the biliary tract
  - Chronic liver disease
- Bilirubin and alkaline phosphatase (ALP) level indicate cholestasis, a blockage of bile flow.
- ALT activity is a measure of the integrity of liver cells or parenchymal liver disease.
- The serum albumin concentration and prothrombin time is a measure of the liver's synthetic capacity.

Table 32.4: Basis and rationale of biochemical tests done in liver disease and jaundice.

No.	Biochemical tests	Basis/Rationale

1.	**Aminotransferases (ALT and AST)**	◆ Raised plasma transaminase concentrations are indicative of hepatocyte damage
		◆ ALT is more specific for liver disease. AST is less widely used in the assessment of liver disease because it is found in other tissues (myocardium, skeletal muscle, brain and kidney) and may rise in acute necrosis of these organs besides liver cell injury
		◆ The activity of ALT is widely used as a sensitive, marker of liver damage due to:
		  » Liver cirrhosis
		  » Hepatitis (hepatic jaundice)
		  » Fatty liver
		  » Liver tumor or cancer
		  » Toxic injury due to drug overdose
		◆ This test is mainly done along with other tests (such as ALP, and bilirubin) to diagnose and monitor liver disease

Contd...

Contd...

No.	Biochemical tests	Basis/Rationale
2.	**Alkaline phosphatase (ALP)**	• Alkaline phosphatase test is often used to diagnose diseases of the liver or bones or type of jaundice • The ALP is produced by many tissues, especially bone, liver, intestine and placenta and is excreted in the bile • Elevation in activity of the enzyme can thus be found in diseases of bone, liver and in pregnancy. In the absence of bone disease and pregnancy, elevated ALP levels generally due to hepatobiliary disease • Increased ALP activity in cholestasis (such as obstructive jaundice) is due to increased synthesis by cells lining the bile canaliculi in response to cholestasis which is regurgitated into plasma • A raised ALP concentration in the presence of a raised γ-glutamyl transpeptidase (GGT) suggests that the ALP is of hepatic origin
3.	**γ-glutamyl transpeptidase (GGT)**	• GGT is derived from the cells of hepatobiliary tract. In response to prolonged intake of alcohol and drugs, such as phenobarbital and phenytoin, synthesis of the enzyme is induced and plasma GGT activity increases • High levels of GGT in the blood may be a sign of **cholestasis** (such as obstructive jaundice) or enzyme induction • Alcohol induces activity of GGT and it is increased by ingestion of alcohol even in absence of liver disease. It can also be used to screen for or monitor alcohol abuse • A GGT test cannot diagnose the specific cause of liver disease. So, it is usually done along with alkaline phosphatase (ALP) test
4.	**Serum bilirubin** • Conjugated or direct bilirubin which is water soluble. • Unconjugated or indirect bilirubin which is water insoluble	• An increase in **serum bilirubin** occurs due to many causes, and results in **jaundice** • Estimation of **direct** and **indirect bilirubin** is useful for the **differential diagnosis of jaundice** • In **hemolytic** jaundice, **unconjugated** bilirubin is increased. Hence, Van den Bergh test is indirect positive • In **obstructive** jaundice, **conjugated** bilirubin is elevated and Van den Bergh test is direct positive • In **hepatic** jaundice, both **conjugated** and **unconjugated** bilirubin are increased hence a biphasic reaction is observed
5.	**Urine bilirubin** Only conjugated bilirubin excreted in urine which is detected by **Fouchet's test**	• In normal individuals, bilirubin is not excreted in the urine. When it is present in the urine, it indicates some disease of the liver or jaundice • In obstructive and hepatic jaundice, conjugated bilirubin appears in urine • In hemolytic jaundice, unconjugated bilirubin is increased in blood; it does not appear in urine • Normally, trace amounts of urobilinogen are present in urine
6.	**Urine Urobilinogen** Urine urobilinogen is estimated semi-quantitatively, by Ehrlich's aldehyde reagent.	• The amount of urobilinogen present in urine depends on the amount of bilirubin entering the intestine. • An increase in urobilinogen in urine is found in hemolytic jaundice due to excess production of bilirubin. • In hepatitis, the urobilinogen in urine may be normal or decreased. • In obstructive jaundice, due to the complete biliary obstruction, bilirubin is unable to enter the intestine and no urobilinogen is found in urine.
7.	**Serum total proteins, albumin and A:G** ratio (globulin is calculated by total proteins minus albumin)	• Albumin is the major serum protein synthesized and secreted by liver • Hypoalbuminemia is a feature of advanced chronic liver disease (such as cirrhosis) as well as in severe acute liver damage • The reversal of the A:G ratio may be seen in conditions hypoalbuminemia or where globulins are abnormally high, e.g., multiple myeloma
8.	**Prothrombin time**	• Prothrombin time is a measure of the activities of certain coagulation factors made by the liver and is used as an indicator of hepatic synthetic function • An increased prothrombin time indicates the failure of hepatic synthesis of one or more of the clotting factors which is an indicator of severity of acute liver disease

BASIS AND RATIONALE OF BIOCHEMICAL TESTS DONE IN PANCREATITIS (TABLE 32.5)

Pancreatitis is inflammation of the pancreas. The two forms of pancreatitis are acute and chronic. Abdominal pain is the major symptom of acute pancreatitis. Pain is more intense when patient is supine and there is relief by sitting with trunk flexed and knees drawn up. Nausea, vomiting, and abdominal distention are also frequent complaints. Physical examination may reveal low-grade fever, tachycardia, and hypotension. USG abdomen and computed tomography (CT) scan abdomen are important diagnostic tests for diagnosing pancreatitis and looking for its complications.

Table 32.5: Basis and rationale of biochemical tests done in pancreatitis.

No.	Biochemical tests	Basis/Rationale
1.	Serum amylase and lipase Both enzymes are secreted by pancreatic acinar cells	• Both enzymes will be elevated due to inflammation or damage to pancreas • Serum lipase the preferred test as it is more specific to pancreas and remains elevated for a longer period compare to amylase

BASIS AND RATIONALE OF BIOCHEMICAL TESTS DONE IN NEPHROTIC SYNDROME

Nephrotic syndrome is not a specific kidney disease. It can occur in any kidney disease that damages the filtering units that allows them to leak protein into the urine. Primary causes of nephrotic syndrome are diseases that affect only the kidneys which damage the glomeruli. Secondary causes of nephrotic syndrome are diseases that affect the whole body, including the kidneys. The most common secondary cause of nephrotic syndrome is diabetes known as diabetic nephropathy.

- ❖ Signs and symptoms of nephrotic syndrome are:
  - Severe swelling (edema), particularly around eyes and in ankles and feet
  - Foamy urine, a result of excess protein in urine
  - Weight gain due to fluid retention
  - Fatigue
  - Loss of appetite
- ❖ The manifestation of nephrotic syndrome includes:
  - Proteinuria (more than 3 g/day)
  - Hypoalbuminemia with plasma albumin less than 3 g/dL and reversed albumin to globulin ratio.
  - Generalised edema
  - Hyperlipidemia which follows lipiduria (lipoprotein also leak across the glomerular wall)
- ❖ Increased permeability of the glomerular membrane result in **massive proteinuria** leading to hypoalbuminemia. The subsequent decreased plasma oncotic pressure causes generalized **edema**. There is also sodium and water retention which aggravate the edema.
- ❖ **Hyperlipidemia:** Most patients with nephrotic syndrome have increased blood levels of cholesterol and triglyceride, LDL, VLDL and decrease in HDL. This is mainly due to impaired clearance and increased lipoprotein biosynthesis.
- ❖ Impaired clearance in nephrotic patients is due to:
  - Decreased hepatic lipase and lipoprotein lipase (LPL) activity decreases catabolism of lipoprotein.
  - Reduced uptake of LDL by liver due to decrease in LDL receptor. Decrease in LDL receptor is due increase in hepatic levels of **proprotein convertase subtilisin kexin type 9 (PCSK9)** which degrades the LDL receptor.
- ❖ Decrease in uptake of LDL by liver leads to a low concentration of intrahepatic free cholesterol. Low concentration of intrahepatic free cholesterol increases the activity of HMG-CoA reductase. In addition, nephrotic syndrome leads to a significant increase in liver acyl-CoA cholesterol acyltransferase (ACAT) activity, which results in enhanced esterification of cholesterol and reduction of intracellular free cholesterol. An increased activity of HMG-CoA (Hydroxy-Methylglutaryl-CoA) reductase and reduction of intracellular free cholesterol leads to an increased endogenous synthesis of cholesterol **(Figure 32.1)**.
- ❖ As well as decreased activity of 7-**hydroxylase** (required for the synthesis of bile acids from cholesterol), results in lower use of cholesterol in the bile acid synthesis and results in an increased concentration of cholesterol causing hypercholesterolemia.

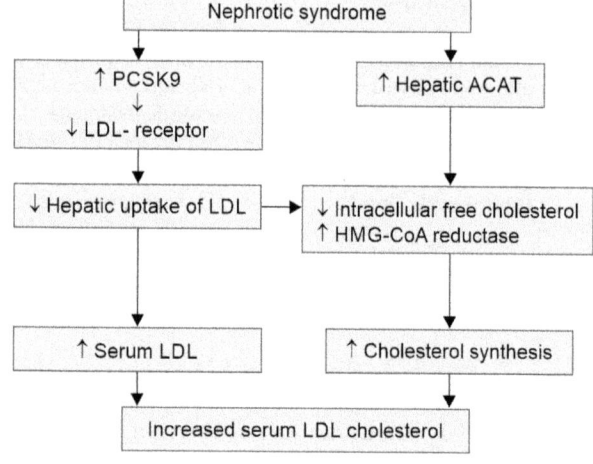

Figure 32.1: Increased blood cholesterol in nephrotic syndrome.

- The reduction in cholesterol uptake caused by LDL receptor deficiency and the reduction in intracellular free cholesterol by ACAT promote activation of **sterol regulatory element-binding protein-2 (SREBP-2)** and **SREBP-1**.
  - Activation of SREBP-2 increases cholesterol synthesis by activating HMG-CoA reductase, that causes hypercholesterolemia. Activation of SREBP-1 increases synthesis of **fatty acids** that causes **hypertriglyceridemia** in nephrotic syndrome. Basis and rationale of biochemical tests done in nephrotic syndrome are given in **Table 32.6**.

Table 32.6: Basis and rationale of biochemical tests done in nephrotic syndrome.

No.	Biochemical Tests	Basis/Rationale
1	Urine protein tests (There are several kinds of urine protein tests)	
	i. Dipstick testing	• Dipstick testing is the most widely used method of screening for proteinuria. The dipstick test can detect the presence of albumin in a sample of urine. It does not provide an exact measurement of albumin • It is convenient for both patient and clinician and provides immediate result at the point of care • However, it gives only a rough indication of the presence or absence of proteinuria and cannot be used alone to diagnose nephrotic syndrome. It must be used in conjunction with more reliable tests.
	ii. 24-hour urine protein test	• This test is performed when there is little protein detected on the dipstick • Urine sample is collected over 24 hours and protein content in the urine over a 24-hour period is estimated. Normally small amount of proteins are present in normal urine (less than 150 mg total protein and 6 mg albumin per day) • An increase in urine protein is a sensitive indicator of kidney disease

	iii. Urine albumin-to-creatinine ratio (UACR)	• Since collection of urine for 24 hours is inconvenient for adults and difficult for infants and children. The specific urine albumin-to-creatinine ratio (UACR) can be determined from a spot random urine sample and is substituted for a 24-hour urine protein measurements
		• The UACR test uses a random single urine sample to estimate the amount of albumin lost in 24 hours. The test measures both albumin and creatinine.
		• Creatinine is a waste product of normal muscle activity which is removed from the body in urine. Total daily creatinine production is relatively constant, so this ratio test is an alternative way to estimate total daily urine albumin level without doing a full 24-hour urine sample
		• UACR is calculated by dividing albumin concentration in milligrams by creatinine concentration in grams
		• An albumin-to-creatinine ratio test is reported in milligrams of albumin per gram of creatine (mg/g) found in one deciliter of urine. This may also be listed in international units measured in milligrams per millimole (mg/mmol)
		• In spot urine specimens, normal level of UACR is below 6 mg/g
		  » The normal UACR value is less than or equal to 17 mg/g in men but in women, the level is observed to be higher ranging around 25 mg/g
		  » Value of 6 to 60 mg/g in the spot urine is considered as presence of microalbuminuria
		• A high concentration of protein in the urine may indicate kidney damage that warrants further investigation

2	Serum proteins	• Serum total protein and albumin levels are decreased due to excretion in urine • When patients become hypoproteinemic and hypoalbuminemic due to excessive proteinuria, the normal balance of oncotic and hydrostatic forces at the capillary level is disturbed, leading to edema which is a common sign of nephrotic syndrome
3	Serum lipid profile	• To detect hypertriglyceridemia and hypercholesterolemia • High levels of both triglycerides and cholesterol in the blood are linked to nephrotic syndrome and may increase the risk of complications such as myocardial infarction.
4	Serum creatinine and blood urea (Renal function test)	• To monitor the overall function of the kidney • They may be normal or increased

BASIS AND RATIONALE OF BIOCHEMICAL TESTS DONE IN PROTEINURIA

Proteinuria is a broad term used to describe abnormal urinary excretion of protein and the protein concentration in the blood falls. Albumin is the protein most likely to appear in the urine, which is why proteinuria is sometimes called **albuminuria**. Persistent proteinuria is a marker of **kidney damage**. Other proteins can also leak into the urine. The level and type of protein reveals the degree of the damage, as well as the risk for developing kidney failure.

When patients become **hypoproteinemic** and **hypoalbuminemic** due to excessive proteinuria, the normal balance of **oncotic** and **hydrostatic forces** at the capillary level is disturbed, leading **edema** (loss of fluid into the interstitial space).

Types of Proteinuria

Glomerular proteinuria: These proteinurias are due to defect in glomerular filtration. Normally, the total amount of protein excreted in urine over 24 hours is **less than 150 mg** and less than **6 mg** of **albumin** and is not detectable by routine tests. The glomeruli of kidney are not permeable to plasma proteins and therefore do not usually allow passage of **albumin.** So plasma proteins are absent in normal urine. Protein in urine is an indicator of **leaky glomeruli** and is the first sign of **glomerular injury** before a decrease in GFR. When the glomeruli are damaged the condition is called **nephritis** or **glomerulonephritis.** Other conditions can lead to nephritis, including hypertension, heart disease and diabetes, as well as other types of kidney disease.

- ❖ Excretion of albumin in the range **6 to 60 mg/day** is termed **microalbuminuria.** Microalbuminuria is the earliest sign of renal damage due to **diabetes mellitus** and **hypertension.**
- ❖ Excretion of albumin more than **60 mg/day** is indicative of significant damage to the glomerular membrane as seen in **nephrotic syndrome** and **diabetic nephropathy.**

Tubular proteinuria: These proteinurias are due to excretion of small molecular weight proteins secreted by tubules, such as α_1-**microglobulin,** β_2-**microglobulin,** and **retinol-binding protein**. If these proteins are detected in excess in the urine, this indicates tubular rather than glomerular dysfunction, i.e., an inability of the renal tubules to reabsorb them.

Overflow proteinuria: This proteinuria occurs when the ability of the glomeruli to retain proteins is overwhelmed by the total quantity of protein in circulation. Usually, they are small proteins, such as light chain fragments of immunoglobulin, seen in **multiple myeloma.** Multiple myeloma involves malignant proliferation of plasma cells which produce light chain fragments of immunoglobulins which are excreted in the urine. These light chain fragments of immunoglobulin called **Bence-Jones proteins.** This type of proteinuria is not detected by dipstick.

Protein is usually first detected by qualitative methods. Persistence of proteinuria requires quantitative estimation which is useful in diagnosis, treatment and follow-up of the patient. **Table 32.7** shows the basis and rationale of biochemical tests done in proteinuria.

Table 32.7: Basis and rationale of biochemical tests done in proteinuria.

No.	Biochemical Tests	Basis/Rationale
1.	**Qualitative tests**	
	i. Heat coagulation test	• This test is based on the principle that proteins get precipitated when boiled in an acidic medium • After heating cloudiness or turbidity indicates the presence of either proteins or phosphates/carbonates • If turbidity remains even after addition of 10% glacial acetic acid means protein is present in urine. If turbidity disappears, that is due to phosphates or carbonates present in urine
	ii. Sulfosalicylic acid test	• Urine appears as a cloudy turbid solution or whitish which indicates that albumin is present in the sample
	iii. Heller's test	• At the intersection of the two layers, a white ring appears which indicates that albumin is present in the given sample of urine
	iv. Dipstick testing	• A positive result indicates an approximate albumin concentration of 6 mg% or more
2.	**Quantitative tests** 24-hour urine protein	*Refer* **Table 32.6**

BASIS AND RATIONALE OF BIOCHEMICAL TESTS DONE IN EDEMA

Edema is defined as accumulation of excess fluid in the interstitial tissue spaces. Generalized edema is termed as **anasarca**. Edema may be caused by:
1. Increased vascular hydrostatic pressure (e.g., heart failure)
2. Decreased colloidal osmotic pressure (oncotic pressure) due to reduced plasma albumin.
   - Decreased synthesis of protein (e.g., liver cirrhosis, protein malnutrition)
   - Increased loss of protein (e.g., nephrotic syndrome)
3. Lymphatic drainage obstruction (e.g., inflammation or neoplasia)
4. Sodium and water retention (e.g., renal failure)

- **Increased hydrostatic pressure** forces large volume of fluid into the interstitial space, which is far in excess of what can be removed by the osmotic pressure of plasma or by the lymphatic drainage. Thus, fluid accumulates causing edema, for example, in patients with congestive heart failure.
- **Decreased osmotic pressure (oncotic pressure)** is due to hypoalbuminemia. Albumin has four times higher plasma oncotic pressure than globulin. Thus mainly hypoalbuminemia (<2.5 g/dL) generally results in edema. Therefore, conditions in which albumin are either lost from the circulation or synthesized in inadequate amounts are common causes of reduced plasma oncotic pressure. For example:
  - In nephrotic syndrome, damaged glomerular capillaries become leaky leading to the loss of albumin; >3.5g/day in the urine and results in generalized edema.
  - Reduced albumin synthesis occurs in liver disease, such as cirrhosis and protein malnutrition (kwashiorkor) due to decreased availability of protein.
- **Lymphatic drainage**: The interstitial fluid is get drained by osmotic pressure as well as some amount also gets drained by the lymphatic system. Thus, obstruction of the lymphatic system leads to accumulation of fluid in the interstitial space called lymphedema. For example:
  - **Filariasis,** a parasitic infection can cause edema of lower extremity due to inflammation of the lymphatics.
  - Complication of **radical mastectomy** (removal of breast along with axillary lymph nodes) for carcinoma of the breast. Removal of axillary lymph nodes leads to obstruction to the lymphatic drainage results in lymphedema of the arm.
- **Sodium and water retention:** Excessive retention of salt can lead to edema by increasing hydrostatic pressure and reducing plasma osmotic pressure. Salt and water retention are caused by **acute renal failure** and **glomerulonephritis.**

Tests Done in Edema

To find out the underlying cause of edema the following diagnostic tests are performed.
- **Urine analysis:** The urinalysis reveals proteinuria in the nephrotic syndrome, and hematuria and casts in the urinary sediment suggest glomerulonephritis.
- **Blood tests**
  - *Kidney function test:* For the screening of renal failure.
  - *Liver function test:* The serum bilirubin and hepatocellular enzymes provide an initial assessment of liver function.
  - *Serum total protein and albumin:* Serum albumin permits a useful estimate of the plasma oncotic pressure
  - *Levels of electrolytes:* An electrolyte imbalance may be a sign of a heart or kidney problem.

BASIS AND RATIONALE OF BIOCHEMICAL TESTS DONE IN RENAL FAILURE

The term renal failure denotes inability of the kidneys to perform excretory function leading to retention of nitrogenous waste products from the blood. Renal failure is classified as:
- Acute renal failure (ARF) and
- Chronic renal failure (CRF) or chronic kidney failure (CKD)
- When a patient needs renal replacement therapy, the condition is called **end-stage renal disease (ESRD).**

Acute Renal Failure (ARF)

In ARF, there is an abrupt deterioration in renal function occurring over a period of hours to days and is usually reversible. ARF arises from a variety of problems affecting the kidneys and/or their circulation. ARF is characterized by an increase in **serum creatinine** and blood **urea** with a **decrease in urine output** and **estimated glomerular filtration rate (eGFR)** over a period of hours or days. ARF may be classified as:

- **Pre-renal**: Due to sudden decrease in blood supply to the nephron which results in depression of GFR. The major causes of pre-renal include inadequate cardiac output and hypovolemia (a decreased volume of circulating blood).
- **Renal**: Due to disease/damage of kidney itself. This may be due to glomerulonephritis or nephrotoxicity.
- **Post-renal**: The urinary drainage of the kidneys is impaired because of a urethral obstruction due to kidney stones or malignancy.

Chronic Renal Failure (CRF) or Chronic Kidney Failure (CKD)

- CKD is characterized by progressive and irreversible deterioration of renal function due to slow destruction of renal parenchyma. The principle manifestations of CKD are:
  - Dehydration
  - Edema
  - Hyperkalemia
  - Metabolic acidosis
  - Hyperphosphatemia
  - Hypercalcemia
  - Anemia
  - Congestive heart failure
- Causes of CKD include:
  - Diabetes mellitus
  - Glomerulonephritis
  - Hypertension
  - Renal calculi
  - Urinary tract obstruction
- In CKD GFR is less than 20% to 25% of normal. The kidneys cannot regulate volume and solute composition, and patient develops edema, metabolic acidosis and hyperkalemia.
- In CKD renal tubules may lose their ability to reabsorb water and so concentrate urine. The impaired ability to regulate salt and water balance may lead to overhydration or dehydration.
- Tubular proteinuria may occur as the result of a tubular defect in the handling of proteins. In tubular proteinuria, less than 2 g/day of protein is excreted.
- As CKD progresses, the ability of the kidneys to reabsorb bicarbonate and excrete hydrogen ions in the urine becomes impaired. Bicarbonate, which is normally completely reabsorbed. As a result of these changes the patient may develop acidosis. The retention of hydrogen ions causes renal tubular acidosis (RTA). RTA is a metabolic acidosis.
- In CKD the renin-angiotensin-aldosterone system is activated resulting in hypertension. Hypertension may leads to cardiac failure.
- The Fanconi syndrome is a group of renal tubular defects that results in glucosuria, aminoaciduria, hypophosphatemia, and renal tubular acidosis.
- Anemia is often associated with CKD due to failure of erythropoietin production from the renal cortex.

Tests Done in Renal Failure

Patients with renal failure have a variety of different clinical presentations. Chronic renal failure results in retention of nitrogenous waste products normally excreted in urine. The reduction in GFR can be detected by measurement of **urea** and **creatinine** in blood or **creatinine clearance**. The estimated GFR (eGFR), a laboratory calculation taking into account the serum creatinine, age, and sex of individual, is now the most common method of reporting renal function in adults. eGFR along with urine albumin content is used to recognize stages of CKD ranging from CKD-1 to CKD-5 **(Table 32.8)**. The key laboratory tests performed in patients with renal failure are given in **Table 32.9**.

- In CKD-1, eGFR is normal but there is other evidence of kidney disease, such as **proteinuria.**
- In CKD-5, eGFR is <15 mL/min per 1.73 m^2.
- Patient with stage—5 are said to have **end stage renal failure**.
- Patient with stage—5 CKD who are being treated by dialysis or have a functioning kidney transplant are said to be on '**renal transplant therapy**'.

Table 32.8: Classification of CKD by eGFR.

Stage of CKD	eGFR result	What it means
Stage 1	90 of higher	• Mild kidney damage • Kidneys work as well as normal
Stage 2	60–89	• Mild kidney damage • Kidneys still work well
Stage 3a	45–59	• Mild to moderate kidney damage • Kidneys do not work as well as they should
Stage 3b	30–44	• Moderate of severe damage • Kidneys do not work as well as they should
Stage 4	15–29	• Severe kidney damage • Kidneys are close to not working al all
Stage 4	less than 15	• Most severe kidney damage • Kidney are very close to not working or have stopped working (failed)

Table 32.9: Basis and rationale of biochemical tests done in renal failure.

No.	Biochemical tests	Basis/Rationale
1.	**Urine analysis:** • Urine volume • Urine creatinine • 24 hour protein • Protein: creatinine ratio • Abnormal parameters » pH » Specific gravity » Proteins » Blood » Ketone bodies » Glucose	• Routine urine examination is usually the first test undertaken to assess the renal function and very often it gives some important information, such as **proteinuria, hematuria** to do further renal investigation. Its analysis, therefore, is important in evaluating kidney function • It may reveal the disease anywhere in the urinary tract • Microscopic examination can identify the presence of urinary casts and crystals. • Urine analysis is therefore more sensitive to changes in renal function, showing abnormal results within the first day of renal dysfunction
2.	**Blood tests** • Blood urea/blood urea nitrogen • Serum creatinine	• Serum **urea** and **creatinine** are markers of renal function. Both these substances are primarily excreted in the urine. Deterioration of renal function is, therefore associated with increases in the serum levels of these substances • Creatinine is considered a better marker of renal function than urea because its blood level is not significantly affected by nonrenal factors, thus making it a specific indicator of renal function • An increase of these end products in the blood is called azotemia
3.	**Clearance test**	• The renal clearance test is performed to measure the glomerular filtration rate (GFR) • GFR provides an index of status of functioning of glomeruli • Lower than normal GFR measurements indicate acute and chronic renal failure • An important drawback associated with the use of clearance tests to estimate GFR is the need for an accurately timed urine sample. However, this problem can be overcome by employing formulae, which can be used to calculate an estimated value for GFR called **eGFR,** using serum creatinine values alone by correcting for age, sex, and body weight

BASIS AND RATIONALE OF BIOCHEMICAL TESTS DONE IN GOUT (TABLE 32.10)

Gout is a clinical syndrome caused by **hyperuricemia** and recurrent **acute arthritis**. The increased serum uric acid is due to either increased formation of uric acid or its decreased renal excretion. It is caused by deposition of monosodium urate crystals in joints that affects the joints and leads to painful arthritis. The kidneys are also affected, since excess urate is also deposited in the kidney tubules (nephrolithiasis) and leads to renal failure. Gout is classified into two broad types:
1. **Primary gout:** In primary gout, increased level of uric acid is associated with increased synthesis of purine nucleotides. Increased synthesis of purine nucleotides is caused by defective enzymes of purine nucleotide biosynthesis.
2. **Secondary gout** results from a variety of diseases that cause:
   - An **elevated destruction of cells** which occurs in **cancers** (leukemia, polycythemia), **psoriasis** and **hypercatabolic states** (starvation, trauma, etc.) or
   - **Decreased elimination of uric acid** which occurs in occurs in **chronic renal disease** due to reduced glomerular filtrate rate.
   - Type-I glycogen storage disease (**Von Gierke's disease**), due to deficiency of **glucose-6-phosphatase.**

Table 32.10: Basis and rationale of biochemical tests done in gout.

No.	Biochemical tests	Basis / Rationale
1.	Serum uric acid	• To diagnose gout and monitor the progress • Elevated levels of uric acid in the blood may be related to gout • A uric acid level in the blood between 3.5 and 7.2 mg/dL is considered normal • However, not all hyperuricemic patients have gout, so further diagnostic tests are recommended in order to proper diagnosis
2.	Urine uric acid	• A uric acid level in the urine between 250 and 750 mg is considered normal • Such as serum uric acid test, urine uric acid test will not be used alone when diagnosing gout • It gives a clue to a gout diagnosis but this test is not conclusive on its own • Low levels of uric acid in urine may be related to kidney disease
3.	Synovial fluid examination	• The most accurate diagnostic test for gout is the examination of synovial fluid, the liquid that surrounds joints and provides them with protection and nutrients • In this, fluid is extracted from the affected joint and observed under the microscope. Urate crystals are found in the synovial fluid

BASIS AND RATIONALE OF BIOCHEMICAL TESTS DONE IN THYROID DISORDERS (TABLE 32.11)

The thyroid gland produces two related hormones, thyroxine (T_4) and Triiodothyronine (T_3). These hormones play major role in metabolism and growth and development of tissues. The thyroid disorders can be divided into two types:
1. **Hyperthyroidism** (due to excess thyroid hormone secretion)
2. **Hypothyroidism** (due to deficient thyroid hormone secretion)

Hyperthyroidism (thyrotoxicosis): Hyperthyroidism causes sustained high plasma concentration of T4 and T3. There is often generalized increase in the metabolic rate and associated with clinical features, such as; heat intolerance, a fine tremor, tachycardia, weight loss, tiredness, anxiety, sweating and diarrhea. Hyperthyroidism is most commonly occurring in Graves' disease.

Hypothyroidism: Hypothyroidism usually develops slowly. An underactive thyroid gland results in hypothyroidism. There is often generalized slowing down of metabolism with lethargy, bradycardia, depression and weakness. Hypothyroidism most commonly occurs in iodine deficiency (most common cause worldwide), Hashimoto's thyroiditis (autoimmune disease due to destruction of thyroid gland).

Table 32.11: Basis and rationale of biochemical tests done in thyroid disorders.

No.	Biochemical tests	Basis/Rationale
1.	Serum TSH	♦ TSH is secreted by anterior pituitary gland and regulates synthesis of thyroid hormones ♦ The level of thyroid stimulating hormone (TSH) is always estimated in all cases of thyroid disorders ♦ Increased levels of serum TSH are seen in primary **hypothyroidism** due to absence of negative feedback control on the pituitary ♦ Decreased levels of serum TSH are associated with: » Primary hyperthyroidism (thyroid gland failure) » Secondary hypothyroidism (anterior pituitary failure) » Tertiary hypothyroidism (hypothalamic failure)
2.	Serum total T_3 and total T_4	♦ Changes in total thyroid hormone concentration are far less sensitive indices of thyroid function than is TSH; for this reason, they should not be measured alone ♦ The concentration of total serum thyroxine can be affected by changes in the concentration of thyroid-binding globulin (TBG), in the absence of thyroid disease. Because more than 99.9% of thyroid hormone is protein bound ♦ Values can be increased in hyperthyroidism, increased concentration of TBG (as in pregnancy and with estrogen therapy) ♦ Values can be decreased in hypothyroidism, decreased concentration of TBG (as in nephrosis due to loss of TBG in urine and in liver disease in which there is a decreased synthesis of TBG)
3.	Serum free T_3 and serum free T_4	♦ Circulatory T_4 and T_3 exist in the free state in the blood, unbound to protein and are more active form ♦ T_3 and T_4 tests are performed depending upon TSH levels ♦ Free thyroid hormone concentration provides more reliable means of diagnosing thyroid dysfunction than measurement of total serum T_4 and T_3 ♦ Increased values are associated with hyperthyroidism and thyrotoxicosis ♦ Decreased values are associated with hypothyroidism
4.	**Thyroid antibodies** ♦ TSH receptor antibodies ♦ Thyroglobulin (Tg) antibodies ♦ Thyroid peroxidase (TPO) antibodies	♦ Autoimmune thyroid diseases produce antibodies against components of thyroid ♦ Several types of antibody against thyroid tissue have been detected in serum of patients with thyroid disease ♦ Measuring these antibodies helps demonstrate the presence of the autoimmune disorders » Graves' disease is commonly associated with the presence of antibodies against the TSH receptor » Hashimoto's thyroiditis is associated with the presence of antibodies against thyroid peroxidase (TPO antibodies, previously called antimicrosomal antibodies) » Measurement of thyroglobulin (Tg) antibody is of particular use in assessing the presence of any remnant thyroid tissue after thyroidectomy, performed for malignancy

BASIS AND RATIONALE OF BIOCHEMICAL TESTS DONE IN DISORDERS OF ACID-BASE BALANCE (TABLE 32.12)

The normal pH of blood is maintained within a remarkable constant level of 7.35 to 7.45.

Acid–base imbalance causes the blood pH to deviate out of the normal range (7.35 to 7.45).

❖ The term **"acidemia"** describes the state of an arterial blood pH <7.35, while **acidosis** is used to describe the pathological conditions leading to these states
❖ The term **"alkalemia"** describes the state of an arterial blood pH >7.45, while **alkalosis** is used to describe the pathological conditions leading to these states
❖ Acid-base disorders are classified, in terms of their immediate cause, as follows:
  - **Metabolic acidosis:** Decrease in bicarbonate (HCO_3^-) concentration
  - **Metabolic alkalosis:** Increase in bicarbonate (HCO_3^-) concentration
  - **Respiratory acidosis:** Increase in pCO_2 or H_2CO_3 concentration
  - **Respiratory alkalosis:** Decrease in pCO_2 or H_2CO_3 concentration
❖ The assessment of acid-base status is usually done by **arterial blood gas (ABG) analyser** which measures blood **pH, pCO_2, pO_2** and **bicarbonate (HCO_3^-).**

SECTION D: Basis and Rationale of Biochemical Tests Done in Various Disorders (SGD)

Table 32.12: Basis and rationale of biochemical tests done in acid-base balance.

No.	Parameter	Basis/Rationale
1.	pH	• In disease, imbalances between the rates of acid formation and excretion can develop resulting in acidosis and alkalosis • Measurement of blood pH determines the presence of acidosis or alkalosis
2.	HCO_3^-	• To assess the type of acidosis and alkalosis • HCO_3 is the bicarbonate level of the blood and the normal range is 22–26 mEq/L • HCO_3^- is calculated from the Henderson-Hasselbalch equation, using the measured values of pH and pCO_2 in whole arterial blood • Any changes in the concentration of bicarbonate (HCO_3^-) accompanied by a change in pH • In metabolic alkalosis, the HCO_3^- level is elevated • In metabolic acidosis, the HCO_3^- level is decreased • If the pH becomes acidic, the kidneys retain HCO_3 to increase the pH. Conversely, if the pH becomes alkalotic, the kidneys excrete more HCO_3, causing the pH to decrease • In respiratory acidosis, kidneys attempt to compensate by increasing reabsorption of HCO_3^- • In respiratory alkalosis, kidneys excrete an increased amount of HCO_3^- to lower the pH
3.	PCO_2	• The normal pCO_2 level is 35–45 mm Hg. CO_2 forms an acid in the blood that is regulated by the lungs by changing the rate or depth of respirations • As the CO_2 level increases, the pH level will decrease • In metabolic acidosis, the lungs try to compensate by more blowing of CO_2 to raise pH • In metabolic alkalosis, the lungs try to compensate by retaining the CO_2 to lower pH
4.	**Serum electrolytes** Sodium Na^+ Potassium K^+ Chloride Cl^- Bicarbonate HCO_3^-	• Acid/base status may alter electrolyte levels critical to a patient's status • In the assessment of acid base disorders, commonly measured electrolytes are serum Na^+, K^+, Cl^- and HCO_3^- from which anion gap is measured. Acid-base disorders are often associated with alterations in the anion gap • The value of anion gap is useful in assessing the acid base status in diagnosing metabolic acidosis and mix acid base disorders. In metabolic acidosis, the anion gap can increase or remain normal depending on the cause of acidosis • Plasma Cl^- estimation may help in two main situations • Hyperchloremia—occurs in normal anion gap metabolic acidosis. Conversely, hypochloremia is seen in metabolic alkalosis due to chronic vomiting

EU GSPR Authorised Reprsentative
Logos Europe, 9 rue Nicolas Poussin
1700, La Rochelle, France
Phone: +33 (0) 6 67 93 73 78
E-mail: contact@logoseurope.eu

www.ingramcontent.com/pod-product-compliance
Ingram Content Group UK Ltd.
Pitfield, Milton Keynes, MK11 3LW, UK
UKHW050458150426
5217IPUK00025B/1739